Creati

The Power Supplement

Melvin H. Williams, PhD
OLD DOMINION UNIVERSITY

Richard B. Kreider, PhD
UNIVERSITY OF MEMPHIS

J. David Branch, PhD
OLD DOMINION UNIVERSITY

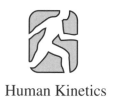

Human Kinetics

Library of Congress Cataloging-in-Publication Data

Williams, Melvin H.
      Creatine : the power supplement / Melvin H. Williams, Richard B. Kreider,
J. David Branch.
      p. cm.
   Includes bibliographical references and index.
   ISBN 0-7360-0162-X
   1. Creatine--Physiological effect. 2. Exercise--Physiological aspects. 3. Sports--
Physiological aspects. 4. Dietary supplements. 5. Athletes. I. Kreider, Richard B.,
1962- II. Branch, J. David, 1956- III. Title.
   QP801.C8 W54 1999
   612´.01575--dc21

                                                           99-21071
                                                            CIP

ISBN **0-7360-0162-X**

Acquisitions Editor: Michael S. Bahrke
Managing Editor: Melinda Graham
Assistant Editor: Laurie Stokoe
Copyeditor: Joyce Sexton
Proofreader: Kathy Bennett
Indexer: Craig Brown
Graphic Designers: Judy Henderson, Nancy Rasmus
Graphic Artist: Judy Henderson
Photo Editor: Clark Brooks
Cover Designer: Jack Davis
Illustrator: Kim Maxey
Printer: Versa Press

QP 801 .C8 W54 1999
Williams, Melvin H.
Creatine

Human Kinetics books are available at special discounts for bulk purchase. Special editions or
book excerpts can also be created to specification. For details, contact the Special Sales Manager
at Human Kinetics.

Printed in the United States of America   10 9 8 7 6 5 4 3 2 1

Web site: http://www.humankinetics.com/

United States: Human Kinetics
P.O. Box 5076
Champaign, IL 61825-5076
1-800-747-4457
e-mail: humank@hkusa.com

Canada: Human Kinetics
475 Devonshire Road Unit 100
Windsor, ON N8Y 2L5
1-800-465-7301 (in Canada only)
e-mail: humank@hkcanada.com

Europe: Human Kinetics, P.O. Box IW14
Leeds LS16 6TR, United Kingdom
+44 (0)113-278 1708
e-mail: humank@hkeurope.com

Australia: Human Kinetics
57A Price Avenue
Lower Mitcham, South Australia 5062
(08) 82771555
e-mail: humank@hkaustralia.com

New Zealand: Human Kinetics
P.O. Box 105-231, Auckland 1
09-523-3462
e-mail: humank@hknewz.com

We are deeply indebted to our loved ones for their patience with and confidence in us.

Jeanne Kruger-Williams and Sara Kruger

Wendy Kreider, Alison Kreider, Ryan Kreider and my parents

Carol Branch, David Powell, and Anne Randolph Powell

Contents

Preface

The two primary determinants underlying successful sport performance are genetic endowment and proper training. To succeed in a given sport at any level of competition, athletes must inherit specific physiologic, psychologic, and biomechanic traits critical to success in that sport, but they must also receive optimal physical, mental, and biomechanical training to maximize this genetic potential. Often, however, in attempts to gain a competitive edge on their opponents, athletes may resort to the use of ergogenic aids, or ergogenics—substances or treatments theoretically designed to improve sports performance beyond the effects of training. In a recent review, Smith and Perry (*Annals of Pharmacotherapy*, 26, 653-59, 1992) indicated athletes view ergogenics as essential components for success.

Throughout history, athletes have used various drugs or hormones to enhance performance, most recently amphetamines, anabolic steroids, human growth hormone, and erythropoietin. However, the use of pharmacological agents to enhance performance, known as doping, has been prohibited by the International Olympic Committee (IOC) and most other athletic governing organizations. Given the increased sophistication of drug testing, most athletes avoid the use of drugs whose detection would be grounds for disqualification.

Thus, athletes continue to search for effective, yet legal, ergogenics. In this regard, as all nutrients are currently legal, the use of dietary supplements marketed as nutritional ergogenics has become increasingly popular. Literally hundreds of dietary supplements, ranging from amino acids to zinc, have been marketed as effective ergogenics to physically active individuals. With several exceptions, such as carbohydrate loading, well-designed research does not support an ergogenic effect of most dietary supplements when added to a healthy, balanced diet. Nevertheless, dietary supplement companies continue to market new products as potential ergogenics. In general, for the vast majority of these dietary supplements, the ergogenic effects have not been evaluated by well-designed research. One major exception is creatine, the subject of numerous studies during the 1990s.

Creatine is a natural dietary constituent of animal foods, but it may also be synthesized from several amino acids by the liver and kidney, so it is not considered to be an essential nutrient. Most creatine is stored in the muscles as free creatine and phosphocreatine (PCr), a high-energy phosphagen important in very high-intensity exercise. About two grams of creatine, normally derived equally from the diet and endogenous synthesis, is needed daily to replenish body stores. However, recent research has investigated whether creatine supplementation, increasing daily dietary intake 20-30 fold, exerts an ergogenic effect on various types of physical performance.

The purpose of this book is to provide a detailed analysis of the effect of creatine supplementation on exercise performance. Chapter 1 defines creatine, providing a brief historical perspective of its evolution as a potential ergogenic aid. Chapter 2 covers normal human creatine requirements, including dietary intake and endogenous synthesis to maintain normal body stores, intestinal absorption and storage in the body, and metabolic functions. Chapter 3 highlights the ergogenic potential of creatine, various supplementation protocols, and the effects of such supplementation on muscle creatine stores, including a summary table indicating the effects on muscle creatine and PCr. Chapter 4 focuses on the major research considerations relative to research conducted with dietary supplements such as creatine. Chapter 5 presents data from both laboratory and field studies evaluating the effect of creatine supplementation to enhance performance in a variety of very high power exercise or sports performance tasks lasting up to 30 seconds. In a similar vein, Chapter 6 focuses on high-intensity exercise or sports performance tasks ranging from 30 to 150 seconds, while Chapter 7 covers similar tasks lasting more than 150 seconds. Chapter 8 presents data evaluating the effect of creatine supplementation in attempts to either gain or lose body mass and favorably modify body composition, including both short-term (less than two weeks) and long-term (14 days or more) supplementation protocols. Chapters 5 to 8 include numerous tables summarizing the key points of studies presented in the respective chapter. Chapter 9 covers health and safety aspects of creatine supplementation, while Chapter 10 discusses legal and ethical issues.

Creatine is one of the most popular dietary supplements ever marketed to a physically-active population. This text represents state-of-the-art information regarding the ergogenic potential and health aspects of creatine supplementation. However, because creatine supplementation has been shown to increase muscular strength and endurance in a number of studies, considerable research attention is being devoted to its possible application to other areas, such as its effects on performance in other types of physical activities and its role in preventing losses of muscle and neural function during aging or with various neuromuscular diseases. Although the findings presented in this text are based on considerable research, future investigations may reveal other possible beneficial applications of creatine supplementation.

Melvin H. Williams, PhD, FACSM

Richard B. Kreider, PhD, FACSM

J. David Branch, PhD, FACSM

Acknowledgments

We would like to express our sincere appreciation to the many athletes, students, coaches, trainers and co-investigators at the University of Memphis and Old Dominion University who have participated in our research over the years in attempts to determine the efficacy and safety of purported ergogenic aids, including creatine supplementation. We would also like to thank our colleagues throughout the world who have contributed their knowledge to the development of this book.

Special thanks to the professionals at Human Kinetics for their continuing involvement in exercise science and sports medicine, particularly to Rainer Martens and Michael Bahrke for their initial encouragement to write this book and to Melinda Graham, our editor, for her patience and understanding during all phases of development. Sincere appreciation is extended to Joyce Sexton, our copy editor who helped us clarify key points in the text. Our gratitude is also extended to Laurie Stokoe, assistant editor, Judy Henderson the graphic artist, and Clark Brooks, the photo editor, for a superb job in enhancing the quality of this presentation.

1

<u>CHAPTER</u>

Introduction

People exercise for various reasons. Some individuals exercise for health, either to prevent the onset of various chronic diseases such as type II diabetes or to rehabilitate the heart from a bout of coronary artery disease. Others exercise to maintain or improve their physical appearance, principally to prevent accumulation of or to lose excess body fat, or to gain muscle mass. Still others exercise in order to compete in sports—their exercise ranging from sporadic exercise training for the fun and enjoyment of recreational sports to daily rigorous exercise training to achieve athletic superiority in highly competitive, organized sports.

No matter what the purpose of exercise, be it improved health, appearance, or sport performance, success is determined by two major factors: genetics and training. Inheritance of specific genetic traits establishes the upper limits in any given individual for the improvement of health, appearance, or athletic ability. In order to maximize this genetic potential, the individual must receive appropriate exercise training.

Athletes at elite levels of sport competition, such as the Olympic Games, have been genetically gifted with physical attributes appropriate for competition in their specific sport, but they have also benefited from expert coaching. At the United States Olympic Training Center and other national Olympic training centers, athletes are exposed to sophisticated training regimens to enhance their physical power, mental strength, and mechanical edge.

Physical power represents the physiological ability to produce energy, or power, specific to the needs of a given sport—be it the explosive power of weight lifting or the prolonged, aerobic endurance power involved in the 42.2K marathon. Mental strength represents the psychological ability to control energy expenditure, that is, to withstand internal or external pressures that may lessen energy control and interfere with optimal energy production, such as the mental anguish associated with lactic acid accumulation in a 400 m dash or the psychological distraction of a jeering audience while one is shooting a basketball free throw. Mechanical edge

1

represents the biomechanical ability to use energy efficiently, or to reduce the physiological energy costs to produce a given amount of power, such as the decreased oxygen cost to run at a given velocity after losing 5 kg of excess body fat. Thus, in order to optimize training, elite athletes may work with sport physiologists to increase physical power, sport psychologists to improve mental strength, and sport biomechanists to obtain a mechanical edge.

Given the technology explosion, many of the training strategies applicable to elite athletes have become available to athletes at all levels of competition, including those in youth sports, those in public schools, colleges, and universities, and those in community leagues and numerous amateur sport organizations such as running and bicycling clubs. With sports becoming increasingly popular each year, literally millions of individuals are involved in competition at various levels. As with elite athletes, genetics and appropriate training are the essential elements for successful performance at various levels of athletic competition—or even for noncompetitive, physically active individuals such as those who engage in vigorous resistance training simply to look and feel better.

At all levels of competition, however, some athletes may believe that they have maximized their training, and in order to improve further they may try to go beyond training to obtain a competitive advantage. In such cases, they may resort to use of ergogenic aids, substances that are theoretically designed to enhance physical power, mental strength, or mechanical edge.

Although athletes have used various purported ergogenics for centuries, only in the past half-century has the use of these aids exploded as sport competition has become more popular and lucrative. In the 1960s and 1970s, the most popular and effective ergogenic aids were drugs, particularly anabolic/androgenic steroids and amphetamines. Anabolic/androgenic steroids were used primarily to increase physical power by increasing muscle mass, whereas amphetamines increased mental strength, and resultant physical power, by stimulating the central and sympathetic nervous systems. However, as drug use in sport increased, causing several deaths in Olympic competition, in 1964 the International Olympic Committee developed legislation banning the use of drugs in sport competition, a practice known as doping. Drug testing, initiated in the 1968 Mexico City Olympic Games, has become increasingly sophisticated over the years, leading to the detection of drug use and resultant expulsion of athletes from Olympic competition. Given the penalties associated with a positive drug test, athletes have become increasingly interested in effective yet legal ergogenic substances, primarily isolated nutrients in foods we eat.

The six major classes of nutrients in the foods we eat are all involved in energy production in one way or another. Although they may have multiple functions related to energy production, carbohydrate and fat primarily provide energy as kilocalories; protein serves as the major foundation for building tissue; vitamins and minerals help regulate energy metabolism; and water is the medium in which energy transformations occur. Although research regarding the effect of various nutrients on energy expenditure has been conducted for over a century, recent advances in nutritional biotechnology as well as in exercise and sport science over the past three decades have stimulated substantial research efforts to explore the potential ergogenic effects of various nutrients and their by-products.

For example, development of the muscle biopsy technique in the late 1960s permitted measurement of muscle glycogen (carbohydrate energy source) during various types of exercise. When it was determined that muscle glycogen was the primary energy source for high-intensity aerobic endurance exercise, such as racing a competitive marathon, various nutritional strategies were studied as a means to increase prerace muscle glycogen levels or to replenish glucose to the muscle during exercise. A quarter-century of research has supported the role of dietary strategies such as carbohydrate loading and glucose replenishment during prolonged exercise. As marathon running became popularized, commercial interests developed unique carbohydrate products such as glucose polymers, or carbohydrate by-products such as pyruvate, in attempts to provide advantages beyond those associated with natural carbohydrate food sources like pasta and rice.

In recent years, hundreds of nutritional, or dietary, supplements have been marketed specifically to athletes. Many of these products—such as energy bars, sports drinks, and protein/amino acid powders—are designed to provide a convenient means by which athletes can obtain calories for optimization of fuel availability before or during exercise, promote resynthesis of energy and anabolism after exercise, and/or increase tolerance to training or effectiveness of recovery from training. In this regard, it is theorized that many of these products provide some ergogenic effect. In addition to the carbohydrate products just mentioned, table 1.1 provides an overview of some specific nutrients that have been studied and marketed for their ergogenic potential. In most cases, research does not support an ergogenic effect for dietary supplements when provided to an athlete who consumes a diet balanced in energy and essential nutrients. However, specific nutrient supplementation may be beneficial to certain athletes under some circumstances, such as carbohydrate loading for marathon running. As another example, the food drug caffeine may be ergogenic for a variety of exercise tasks. The current hottest-selling dietary supplement marketed to sport and exercise enthusiasts as a potential ergogenic is creatine, a nutrient found naturally in various foods.

Creatine is a nutrient found naturally in various foods.

Brief History

Creatine has been recognized as a food constituent for over 150 years, and important historical points have been documented in earlier general reviews (Hunter 1928), as well as more recent reviews, establishing a historical relationship to exercise or sport performance (Balsom et al. 1994; Ekblom 1996; Newsholme and Beis 1996).

Table 1.1 Major Categories of Nutritional Supplements Studied for Their Ergogenic Potential.

Megadoses of essential nutrients

  Carbohydrates and carbohydrate by-products

    Fructose 1,6 diphosphate

    Glucose polymers

    Polylactate

  Lipids and lipid by-products

    Medium-chain triglycerides

    Omega-3 fatty acids

  Protein and amino acids

    Arginine, ornithine, lysine

    Aspartates

    Branched-chain (Leucine, isoleucine, valine)

    Glutamine

    Glycine

    Tryptophan

  Vitamins

    B-complex

      Thiamin (B_1)

      Riboflavin (B_2)

      Niacin

      Pyridoxine (B_6)

      Cyanocobalamin (B_{12})

      Folacin

      Pantothenic acid

    Antioxidants

      Beta carotene

      Vitamin C

      Vitamin E

    Vitamin B_{15}

Minerals

    Boron

    Chromium

    Iron

    Phosphate

    Selenium

    Vanadium

Water

Nonessential nutrients

    Carnitine (L-carnitine)

    Choline

    Coenzyme Q_{10} (Ubiquinone)

Engineered metabolic byproducts of essential nutrients

    CLA (Conjugated linoleic acid)

    DHAP (Dihydroxyacetone pyruvate)

    FDP (Fructose diphosphate)

    HMB (β-hydroxy-β-methylbutyrate)

Plant extracts (phytochemicals)

    Bee pollen

    Gamma oryzanol (Ferulic acid, FRAC)

    Ginkgo biloba

    Ginseng

    Octacosanol

    Smilax officianalis

    Wheat germ oil

    Yohimbine (Yohimbe)

Drug nutrients

    Alcohol

    Alkaline salts

    Caffeine

    Ephedrine, ephedra (Ma Huang)

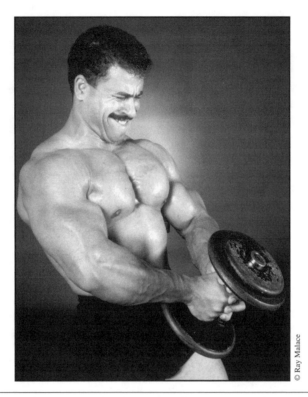

Figure 1.1 Creatine is a popular dietary supplement among those who desire to increase muscle mass.

The following represent several of the salient historical points gleaned from these reviews.

> Creatine has been recognized as a natural substance for over 150 years, but only recently has it been studied extensively in order to evaluate its potential as an ergogenic aid for exercise and sport performance.

Creatine was discovered in 1832 by a French scientist, Michel Eugene Chevreul, who extracted from meat a new organic constituent and named it creatine. Justus von Liebig, in 1847, confirmed that creatine was a regular constituent of animal flesh and reported greater creatine content in wild animals as compared to captive animals that may have been less physically active. In the mid-1880s, creatinine was discovered in the urine, and later authors speculated that creatinine was derived from creatine and was related to total muscle mass. Because extraction of creatine from fresh meat was an expensive process, early research was limited; but nevertheless, even in the early 1900s, creatine supplementation was shown to increase muscle creatine content in animals. Phosphocreatine (PCr), the phosphorylated form of creatine, was discovered in 1927, with observations that it was involved in exercise energy expenditure. Creatine kinase, the enzyme that catalyzes PCr, was discovered in 1934. In 1968, with the discovery of the needle biopsy technique to extract human muscle samples, Swedish investigators examined the role of PCr during exercise and recovery. More recently, nuclear magnetic resonance techniques, which are noninvasive, have been used to study PCr dynamics during exercise.

Creatine was discovered in 1832.

Glycine is one of three amino acids used in the formation of creatine, and gelatin is composed of approximately 25% glycine. As early as 1940, it was theorized that gelatin supplementation possesses ergogenic potential, possibly by increasing muscle PCr levels. Several researchers investigated the ergogenic potential of gelatin or glycine supplementation during the period from 1940 to 1964. Some early, poorly controlled studies provided evidence of a beneficial effect on performance, but more contemporary, well-controlled studies revealed no significant ergogenic effect (Williams 1985).

Research on the potential medical effects of creatine or PCr supplementation, conducted in the 1970s and 1980s, provided some anecdotal evidence that creatine might be an effective ergogenic aid. For example, Sipilä et al. (1981) were investigating the effect of prolonged creatine supplementation on gyrate atrophy of the choroid and retina within the eye, an autosomal-recessive disease often accompanied by clinical findings of mild but morphologically marked progressive atrophy of the type II skeletal muscle fibers. Anecdotally, some patients reported a subjective impression of increased strength during treatment, and one active older runner beat his former record in a 100 m sprint (17 sec vs. 15 sec).

Creatine is a popular dietary supplement among public school, college, Olympic, and professional athletes; one estimate is that 80% of the athletes at the 1996 Summer Olympics in Atlanta used creatine.

Plisk and Kreider (1999) cite anecdotal information of creatine use by athletes in Eastern European block countries as early as the 1960s. Other anecdotal reports emanating from England in the early 1990s suggested that creatine supplementation might benefit sport performance. Two Olympic champions in the 1992 Barcelona Summer Olympic Games, Linford Christie in the men's 100 m dash and Sally Gunnell in the women's 400 m hurdles, reportedly used creatine supplements, as did the Cambridge University rowing team in training for three months before defeating heavily favored Oxford (Associated Press 1993).

Two Olympic champions in the 1992 Barcelona Summer Olympic
Games may have benefited from use of creatine supplements.

Recent newspaper accounts (Duarte 1998; Strauss and Mihoces 1998) indicate
that creatine is a popular dietary supplement among Olympic and professional
athletes. One researcher at Pennsylvania State University estimated that 80% of the
athletes at the 1996 Summer Olympics in Atlanta used creatine. A recent *USA Today*
survey of 115 professional teams showed that of the 71 teams responding, 21
explicitly disapprove of creatine use while 16 approve (Strauss and Mihoces 1998).
The others have no formal position, leaving the decision to the individual players.
Twenty-four teams provide creatine to their athletes. Many celebrated professional
athletes acknowledge creatine use, including Mark McGwire, who recently broke
the home run record for a single season with a total of 70.

Research in the '70s and '80s on the potential medical effects of
creatine or PCr supplementation, provided some anecdotal evidence that creatine might be an effective ergogenic aid.

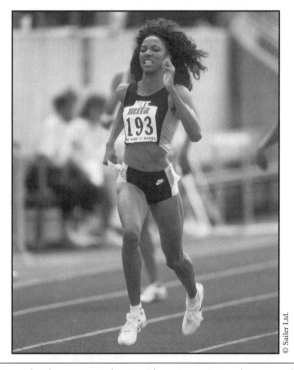

© Sailer Ltd.

Figure 1.2 Anecdotal reports indicate Olympic sprinters have used creatine in
attempts to enhance performance.

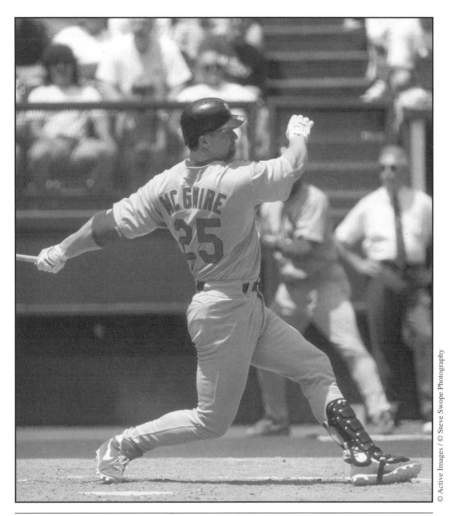

Figure 1.3 Some professional athletes contend that creatine may be used to improve performance.

"There's no magic bullet out there. But creatine is about the closest thing," says Rob Zatchetka, New York Giants offensive lineman and Rhodes scholar finalist with a degree in biochemistry (Strauss and Mihoces 1998).

Creatine also appears to be a popular dietary supplement among college athletes. Costley et al. (1998) recently surveyed anonymously 339 National Collegiate Athletic Association Division IA male and female athletes, representing 14 sports, concerning their level of familiarity with and the perceived benefits or problems associated with the use of various nutritional supplements. Among supplements that respondents considered "most helpful" to their athletic performance, creatine was one of the most frequently cited.

> Creatine appears to be a popular dietary supplement among college athletes and other groups involved in resistance-exercise training.

Creatine supplements are also used extensively by other groups involved in resistance-exercise training. Schneider et al. (1998) reported that U.S. Navy Seals use nutritional supplements mainly to increase muscle mass, strength, and power and that creatine is one of the five most commonly used supplements. Obtaining survey data from nearly 1300 readers of *Muscle Media,* a magazine targeted to weight lifters and bodybuilders, Johnson (1998) presented some interesting demographics about users of creatine monohydrate. The following are highlights of this survey conducted in 1997; the percentages have a ± 3% margin of error.

93.3% of respondents exercised three to six times per week.

92.8% of respondents regularly lifted weights.

96.7% of respondents were male.

61.7% of respondents were between the ages of 21 and 35. The average age was 32.

79.8% of respondents attended or graduated from college.

13.7% of respondents (the highest percentage) listed their profession as "Professional."

40.1% of respondents had an annual salary over $50,000.

40.7% of respondents spent between $51 and $100 a month on nutritional supplements.

48.4% of respondents spent $101 to over $200 a month on nutritional supplements.

> Survey data indicate that most creatine users are male, are between the ages of 21 and 25, have attended or graduated from college, and have a substantial income.

Manufacturers of dietary supplements for athletes are marketing creatine worldwide. SKW Trostberg, a leading manufacturer of creatine, estimates worldwide consumption at 2.7 million kg per year (SKW Trostberg 1998). In the United States, the most recent estimate of sales revenue is $100 million per year (Strauss and Mihoces 1998).

> Manufacturers of dietary supplements for athletes have sales revenues in excess of $100 million per year.

These anecdotal and demographic data suggest that the dietary supplement, creatine, may provide an ergogenic benefit to some athletes. However, one of the problems with the use of dietary supplements, particularly for athletes attempting to achieve a competitive edge, is the belief that if a little is good, a lot is great. Thus, some athletes may misuse dietary supplements and suffer some adverse health consequences. For example, Derek Bell, an outfielder for the Houston Astros, contended that his misuse of creatine supplements may have contributed to kidney ailments that hospitalized him (Duarte 1998). Indeed, the National Football League Tampa Bay Buccaneers distributed a position paper on creatine to all their players, indicating that creatine supplementation may predispose them to such problems as muscle cramping and heat-related illnesses (Strauss and Mihoces 1998). Nevertheless, perceived health risks may not deter some athletes from supplementing with creatine. For example, Rob Zatchetka, New York Giants offensive lineman, knows that there might be potential hazards of creatine use over the long term but says, "I'm willing to use it" (Strauss and Mihoces 1998).

Chapter Summary

Although creatine has been recognized as a natural substance for over 150 years, Ekblom in 1996 indicated that serious research regarding the potential ergogenic effect of creatine supplementation had been implemented only in 1992. However, numerous studies have been conducted in the intervening years in order to evaluate the effect of creatine supplementation on exercise and sport performance, and some limited data are available relative to its effects on various aspects of health. Additionally, numerous reviews (Balsom et al., 1994; Clark, 1997; Greenhaff, 1995; Juhn and Tarnopolsky, 1998A; Kraemer and Volek, 1998; Ööpik et al., 1995; Volek, 1997; Williams and Branch, 1998) evaluating the ergogenic effects of creatine supplementation have been published, but detailed coverage in these reviews is limited because journal publishers normally restrict the number of pages.

The purpose of this book is to provide a comprehensive review of the scientific literature dealing with creatine supplementation and its effects on exercise performance and, where data are available, on health status.

2

CHAPTER

Creatine Requirements and Metabolic Functions

Creatine (methylguanidine-acetic acid), a nitrogenous amine, is a naturally occurring constituent found in food. Although not an essential nutrient, because body needs may be satisfied by endogenous synthesis, creatine nevertheless is intimately involved in human metabolism. This chapter focuses on normal dietary requirements and metabolic functions of creatine.

Creatine, a nitrogenous amine, is a naturally occurring dietary constituent.

Daily Creatine Requirements

Creatine is found naturally in vertebrates, participating in metabolic reactions within the cells and eventually being catabolized in the muscle to creatinine and excreted by the kidneys. In humans, total creatine stores approximate 120 g in the average-sized adult male (70 kg), with correspondingly smaller and larger amounts in individuals who weigh less or more. The daily turnover rate of creatine to creatinine has been estimated to be about 1.6% of the total creatine pool (Balsom et al. 1995; Hoberman et al. 1948). Based on measurements of renal excretion of creatinine, the daily requirement for creatine supplied through the diet or from endogenous synthesis in a 70 kg man approximates 2 g/day (Walker 1979). It should be noted, however, that since many athletes are larger than 70 kg and since intense training promotes protein degradation, serving to increase serum and urinary creatinine levels, larger athletes undergoing intense training may have a greater daily creatine turnover and requirement (e.g., 2 to 3 g/day). There is currently no recommended dietary allowance for creatine because creatine may be synthesized in the body, as discussed later in this chapter.

The daily requirement for creatine supplied through the diet or from endogenous synthesis in a 70 kg man is estimated to be approximately 2g/day.

Dietary Sources of Creatine

Walker (1979) indicated that creatine occurs in vertebrates but has not been found in plants or microorganisms, and since creatine concentrates primarily in muscle tissue, the primary dietary sources of creatine are fish and red meat. However, Balsom et al. (1994) indicted that trace amounts may be found in some plants. As noted in table 2.1, creatine concentration is much higher in animal flesh. For example, there are about 3 to 5 g of creatine per kilogram of uncooked fish (tuna, salmon, cod) and meat (beef, pork). Herring contains about 6 to 10 g of creatine per kilogram. However, the cooking process may degrade some of the creatine found in food. Consequently, the amount of creatine available from dietary sources in omnivorous individuals may be lower depending on the method of food preparation.

The primary dietary sources of creatine are fish and red meat, approximating 3 to 5 g of creatine per kilogram uncooked fish (tuna, salmon, cod) and meat (beef, pork). In strict vegetarians, or vegans, daily creatine intake is virtually zero, and endogenous synthesis is their only source of creatine.

Dietary Intake

Dietary creatine intake may vary considerably. In strict vegetarians, or vegans, daily creatine intake is virtually zero, and endogenous synthesis is the only source of creatine (Greenhaff 1997a). Individuals who consume a normal omnivorous diet, whose protein intake ranges between 1 and 2 g/kg body weight daily, obtain between 0.25 and 1 g/day of creatine from their diet. Although it is possible to increase dietary intake of creatine by consuming more foods rich in creatine (see table 2.1), it would be very difficult to obtain more than 3 to 4 g/day of creatine from dietary sources unless an individual ingested large amounts of protein, such as 1 or more pounds of fish or red meat.

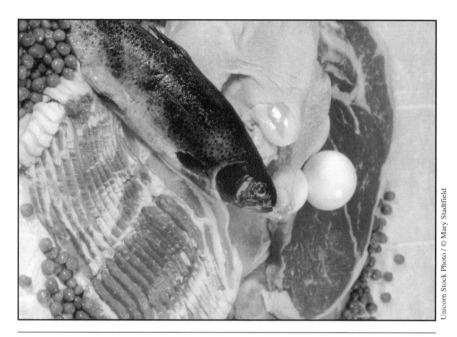

Unicorn Stock Photo / © Mary Stadtfield

Figure 2.1   Meat and fish are the major natural dietary sources of creatine.

Table 2.1   Creatine Content in Selected Foods.

| | Creatine content | |
Food	g/lb	g/kg
Shrimp	Trace	Trace
Cod	1.4	3
Tuna	1.8	4
Salmon	2	4.5
Herring	3-4.5	6.5-10
Beef	2	4.5
Pork	2.3	5
Cranberries	0.01	0.02
Milk	0.05	0.1

Adapted, by permission, from P. Balsom, K. Soderlund, and B. Elkblom, 1994, "Creatine in humans with special reference to creatine supplementation," *Sports Medicine* 18: 268-280.

For individuals who desire to increase dietary creatine intake, commercial supplements containing pure creatine have been developed. Creatine-supplementation protocols are discussed in chapter 3.

Intestinal Absorption of Creatine

Studies indicate that orally consumed creatine is absorbed intact from the intestinal lumen and then enters the bloodstream. This is true despite the presence of highly acidic gastrointestinal secretions during the digestive process (Clark 1996; Syllum-Rapoport et al. 1980). Initial evidence reported by Chanutin (1926) indicated that absorption of creatine from the alimentary tract appeared to be complete and that there was no evidence of acidic and/or bacterial destruction in the intestine. Subsequent studies that have evaluated the metabolic fate of creatine supplementation, as discussed in chapter 3, support these findings.

> Orally ingested creatine is absorbed intact from the intestinal lumen and then enters the bloodstream, and absorption appears to be complete.

Tissue Uptake of Creatine

Following intestinal absorption of creatine, plasma creatine is delivered to various body tissues, including the heart, smooth muscles, brain, and testes; however, as noted later, the vast majority of the body stores of creatine are located in the skeletal muscles. The cellular concentration of creatine is determined by the cell's ability to assimilate creatine from the plasma because there is no muscle synthesis (Clark 1998). In a recent review, Greenhaff (1997b) indicated that two mechanisms have been proposed to explain the very high creatine concentration within skeletal muscle. The first involves the transport of creatine into muscle by a specific sodium-dependent saturable entry process, and the second entails the trapping of creatine within muscle.

> Following intestinal absorption of creatine, plasma creatine is delivered to various body tissues, including the heart, smooth muscles, brain, and testes; however, the vast majority of the body stores of creatine are located in the skeletal muscles. There is evidence that creatine uptake into tissue may also be mediated by insulin.

Early studies demonstrated that creatine entry into muscle occurs actively against a concentration gradient, possibly involving creatine interacting with a specific membrane site that recognizes part of the creatine molecule (Greenhaff 1997b). Radda (1996) indicated that the total creatine content of muscle cells is controlled by an active creatine uptake in which beta 2-receptor stimulation and the activity of sodium-potassium adenosinetriphosphatase (ATPase) play a significant role. Creatine is actively transported into tissues by a sodium-dependent transporter (i.e., two sodium molecules are transported for every creatine molecule), and Clark et al. (1996b) indicate that this transporter is highly specific for creatine.

There is evidence that creatine uptake into tissue may also be mediated by insulin, as suggested by in vitro isolated rat muscle studies (Haughland and Chang 1975). In humans, Green et al. (1996a) reported that ingesting large amounts of carbohydrate (95 g) with creatine (5 g) facilitated greater creatine uptake than ingesting creatine alone. The greater creatine uptake was apparently mediated by a glucose-stimulated release of insulin.

Muscle creatine content is rather stable. Extracellular creatine is sequestered into the cytosol, where rapid phosphorylation by creatine kinase takes place (Clark et al. 1996a). About 60-70% of the muscle total creatine exists in the form of phosphocreatine (PCr) that is unable to pass through membranes, thus trapping creatine in the cell (Greenhaff 1997b). However, creatine may possibly bind to intracellular components, another factor that may facilitate muscle creatine retention (Walker 1979).

Muscle creatine content is rather stable. About 60-70% of the muscle total creatine exists in the form of PCr that is unable to pass through membranes.

Creatine is an osmotically active substance; thus an increase in intracellular creatine concentration may likely induce the influx of water into the cell (Volek et al. 1997a)—an important consideration in relation to body mass and fat-free mass as discussed in chapter 8.

Creatine is an osmotically active substance; thus an increase in intracellular creatine concentration may induce water influx into the cell.

Endogenous Synthesis

Dietary creatine intake accounts for about half of the body's daily need for creatine. The remainder is obtained through endogenous creatine synthesis. Specifically, when dietary availability of creatine is insufficient to meet daily needs, the remaining creatine is synthesized from the amino acids glycine, arginine, and methionine. The entire glycine molecule is incorporated into creatine, whereas arginine furnishes only its amidino group, and methionine its methyl group (Walker 1979).

Creatine is not considered an essential nutrient because it can be synthesized in the body from amino acids.

In humans, the liver appears to be the major site of de novo creatine synthesis (Walker 1979), but the kidney and pancreas may also synthesize creatine (refer to figure 2.2). The first step in creatine synthesis involves the reversible transfer of an amidine group from arginine to glycine to form guanidinoacetic acid. This is followed by an irreversible transfer of a methyl group from S-adenosylmethionine to guanidinoacetic acid, forming creatine.

Walker (1979) indicates that creatine biosynthesis is regulated so as to not interfere with the other metabolic needs of arginine, glycine, and methionine. Arginine participates in the urea cycle; glycine is a precursor of purine nucleotides, which occur in adenosine triphosphate (ATP), deoxyribonucleic acid (DNA), and ribonucleic acid (RNA); and methionine contributes its methyl group to numerous methylations, including synthesis of choline and methylation of DNA and RNA. Creatine biosynthesis is normally controlled by the amidinotransferase, rather than the methyltransferase, reaction.

Creatine synthesis may be modified by various factors. When dietary availability of creatine is low, endogenous synthesis of creatine is increased to maintain normal levels. Thus, vegans must synthesize all their creatine requirements. In humans, dietary gelatin or arginine plus glycine increases biosynthesis (Walker 1979). On the other hand, fasting and increased dietary creatine intake, particularly of creatine

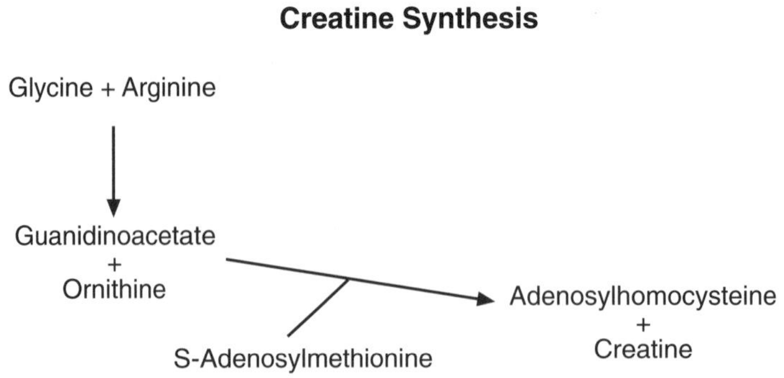

Creatine Synthesis

Figure 2.2 Biochemical pathway of creatine synthesis.
Reprinted, by permission, from R. Kreider, 1998, "Creatine Supplementation: Analysis of ergogenic value, medical safety and concerns," *JEP Online* 1(1).

supplements, will lower amidinotransferase levels in the liver, suppressing synthesis. In fasting, individuals do not need creatine because of decreases in muscle mass, while creatine feeding may suppress creatine synthesis because it simply is not needed (Walker 1979).

Storage in the Body

The body stores creatine in both free and phosphorylated forms. Adding the amounts of phosphorylated and free creatine together yields the total body creatine content (TCr). The average-sized adult male (70 kg) stores about 120 g of creatine. About 95% of the body's creatine is stored in skeletal muscle. Of this amount, about 60-70% binds to phosphate, forming PCr, while the remaining 30-40% remains as free creatine. However, there are differences in the concentrations within various muscle fiber types, as biceps white muscle has 31% more PCr than soleus red muscle (Clark et al. 1996b). The remaining amount of total body creatine (about 5%) is found primarily in the heart, smooth muscles, brain, and testes. Most research has focused on skeletal muscle creatine content.

The body stores creatine in both free and phosphorylated forms (PCr). Adding the amounts of PCr and free creatine together yields the TCr. About 95% of the body's creatine is stored in skeletal muscle, with higher concentrations in fast-twitch muscle fibers. Total creatine stores approximate 120 g in the average-sized adult male (70 kg), with correspondingly smaller and larger amounts in individuals who weigh less or more.

Muscle creatine content is usually expressed as millimoles per kilogram of dry mass or matter (dm). The total creatine content in striated muscle is about 30 mmol/kg (Clark 1997). As 1 mmol of creatine approximates 131 mg, creatine content in muscle approximates 4 g/kg. When muscle biopsies are used to determine creatine concentration, the muscle is usually snap-frozen in liquid nitrogen, freeze-dried, powdered, and then analyzed and reported as creatine per kilogram dm (Harris et al. 1992). Muscle is approximately three-quarters water, so normal total creatine concentrations approximate 120 millimoles per kilogram dm (mmol/kg dm).

Muscle creatine content is usually expressed as millimoles per kilogram of muscle (mmol/kg) and averages about 30 mmol/kg in wet muscle and approximately 120-125 mmol/kg dry muscle, or mass.

On a normal diet, muscle TCr is approximately 120-125 mmol/kg dm. Even strict vegetarians have muscle concentrations approaching normal levels (Harris et al. 1992). In their research with creatine loading, Harris and his colleagues (1992) indicated that a concentration of 155 mmol/kg dm may represent an upper limit for the total creatine pool, at least with the use of their supplementation protocol. Other investigators suggest 160 mmol as an upper limit, but as noted in chapter 3, some individuals exceed this value.

Metabolic Functions

There are several important metabolic functions of creatine that help explain its potential ergogenic value, as will be discussed in chapter 3, and its possible role in relation to various health conditions, discussed in chapter 9. The following discussion deals with the basic role of creatine in energy metabolism important for exercise and sport performance; it also focuses briefly on other functions of creatine in the myocardium and nervous system and in protein synthesis that may have health or sport performance implications.

Energy Metabolism

All cells use ATP as the immediate energy source. The energy needed to facilitate maximal-effort exercise is primarily derived from ATP stored in the muscle. Energy is liberated as the phosphate from ATP is enzymatically removed by an ATPase leaving adenosine diphosphate (ADP) and inorganic phosphate (Pi), as illustrated by the following formula:

$$ATP \leftrightarrow ADP + Pi$$

All cells use ATP as the immediate energy source, but since ATP stores are limited they must be regenerated by other metabolic processes in the cells in order to sustain high muscle power output.

However, Sahlin (1986), discussing differences between endogenous energy sources as to the relative ATP production from each store, indicated that energy derived from ATP stores was limited. Sahlin calculated the available energy capacity (mol ATP), maximal ATP power produced (per mmol ATP/kg dm), exercise intensity supported, and duration of activity allowed per energy source. With regard to anaerobic sources, ATP stores contain approximately 0.02 mol ATP, produce 11.2 mmol ATP kg dm, support very high exercise intensities, and last only approximately 1 to 2 sec.

Although cellular ATP stores are limited, they may be regenerated by other metabolic processes in the cells, including anaerobic glycolysis and oxidative metabolism (Ma et al. 1996). For example, Sahlin (1986) calculates that anaerobic glycolysis contains 5.2 mmol ATP, produces 5.2 mmol ATP kg of dm, supports high-intensity rather than very high intensity exercise, and lasts approximately 7 min. ATP is generated more slowly from oxidative processes.

During very high intensity exercise, the phosphate from the PCr is cleaved off to provide energy for resynthesis of ATP as follows: PCr + ADP $\leftrightarrow$ ATP + Cr. The energy derived from the degradation of PCr allows the ATP pool to be turned over several dozen times during an all-out maximal-effort exercise.

Of interest to this discussion is the role of PCr in ATP generation during intense exercise. Creatine (Cr) is essential to this process in that about two-thirds of the creatine stored in the muscle is phosphorylated by the enzyme creatine kinase (CK) to form PCr. During explosive exercise, the phosphate from the PCr is cleaved off to provide energy for resynthesis of ATP as follows:

$$PCr + ADP \leftrightarrow ATP + Cr$$

Collectively, ATP and PCr energy sources are known as the phosphagen energy system.

The energy derived from the degradation of PCr allows the ATP pool to be turned over several dozen times during an all-out maximal-effort exercise. Sahlin (1986) calculates that PCr stores contain 0.34 mol ATP, produce 8.6 mmol ATP/kg dm, and support very high exercise intensities that are reported to last no more than about 30 sec. However, PCr stores may be more important for shorter-duration maximal tasks, possibly 5-10 sec (Newsholme and Beis 1996). The rate of production of ATP may decrease with time. Greenhaff (1995), citing some of his previous research with Eric Hultman, indicated that PCr utilization begins to decline after only 1.28 sec of contraction, while the corresponding rate from glycolysis does not peak until after about 3 sec of contraction. Greenhaff notes that there appears to be a progressive decline in the rates of ATP provision from both PCr and glycolysis after their initial peak rates, giving the following data regarding ATP production (mmol ATP/sec/kg dm) from PCr:

0-1.3 sec = 9.0
0-2.6 sec = 7.5
0-5 sec = 5.3
0-10 sec = 4.2
10-20 sec = 2.2
20-30 sec = 0.2

> Although there is about three to four times more PCr in the muscle
> than there is ATP, its supply is also limited and needs replenishment
> in order to maintain very high intensity exercise.

Phosphocreatine serves as a temporary energy buffer during periods of intense muscle contraction, when ATP consumption exceeds synthesis (van Deursen et al. 1993). Although there is about three to four times more PCr in the muscle than there is ATP, its supply is also limited and needs replenishment in order to maintain very high intensity exercise. In order to explore the role of PCr and its resynthesis in muscle energetics, a brief review of the enzyme creatine kinase is necessary.

> Phosphocreatine serves as a temporary energy buffer during peri-
> ods of muscle contraction, when ATP consumption exceeds syn-
> thesis.

Creatine Kinase and Energy Production

Walker (1979) indicated that there is only one known enzymatic reaction present in vertebrate tissues for which creatine and PCr are substrates, and that is the reversible reaction catalyzed by creatine kinase (CK).

$$PCr + ADP \leftrightarrow ATP + Cr$$

> There is only one known enzymatic reaction, a reversible reaction
> catalyzed by CK, for which creatine and CPr are substrates: PCr +
> ADP ↔ ATP + Cr.

Evolutionary processes have selected the CK reaction to provide a device for increasing the capacity factor without diminishing the intensity factor. Creatine kinase occurs in extremely high concentrations in muscle and nerve tissues in order to handle high metabolic fluxes during periods of increased energy utilization and generation. At intracellular sites of energy utilization, the reaction is driven to the right by removal of ATP; at sites of energy generation, the reaction is driven to the left by removal of ADP (Walker 1979). Creatine kinase functions as an important cellular enzyme facilitating energy transduction in muscle cells by catalyzing the reversible transfer of a phosphate moiety between ATP and PCr (Clark et al. 1996a).

Creatine kinase exists in various isoforms, and they function simultaneously to form a rapid interconversion of PCr and ATP, which maintains an equilibrium in the muscle. Creatine kinase is composed of two subunit types (M and B isoenzymes, so named because they were first characterized in muscle and brain, respectively), giving three isoenzymes, MM-CK, MB-CK, and BB-CK. In addition, a fourth CK isoenzyme (Mi-CK) is located on the outer side of the inner mitochondrial membrane (Clark 1997; Clark et al. 1996a).

Of interest to this discussion are the MM-CK and Mi-CK isoforms, which are compartmentalized in muscle tissue (Ma et al. 1996). Skeletal muscle is the tissue with the greatest CK activity, and the skeletal muscle CK exists almost exclusively in the MM form. MM-CK, also referred to as myofibrillar CK, is bound to the myofibrils and localized to the A-bands as well as being distributed across the entire filament. MM-CK generates ATP from ADP. Mi-CK is found on the outer surface of the inner mitochondrial membrane and is functionally coupled to oxidative phosphorylation. Mi-CK, at the site of oxidative mitochondrial ATP generation, catalyzes the phosphorylation of creatine to PCr (Clark 1996; Ma et al. 1996). Fast-twitch fibers have greater CK activity, containing a large amount of MM-CK, than slow-twitch oxidative fibers; but the latter have a higher percentage of Mi-CK (Clark 1996; van Deursen et al. 1993).

From an ergogenic viewpoint, resynthesis of PCr could be the critical factor during sustained very high intensity exercise. Although the mechanisms are not clearly understood (Newsholme and Beis 1996), a creatine phosphate shuttle may be the functional mechanism (Ma et al. 1996). In addition to its role as an energy buffer, it has been proposed that the CK-PCr system functions in energy transport on the basis of the functional and physical association of CK isoenzymes with subcellular sites of ATP production and hydrolysis. In this creatine phosphate shuttle concept, PCr and creatine act as shuttle molecules between these sites (van Deursen et al. 1993). One proposed shuttle is believed by some to be functionally coupled to glycolysis (van Deursen et al. 1993), but others believe that the rapid resynthesis of PCr is likely to be oxidative in origin (Blei et al. 1993; Clark 1996; Radda 1996). Mi-CK promotes the formation of PCr from creatine and from ATP formed via oxidative metabolism in the mitochondria (Ma et al. 1996). Phosphocreatine is presumed to diffuse from the mitochondria to the myofibrillar M-band, where it locally serves to replenish ATP with MM-CK as catalyzing agent (van Deursen et al. 1993). Finally, creatine diffuses back to sites of ATP synthesis for rephosphorylation (see figure 2.3).

From an ergogenic viewpoint, resynthesis of PCr could be the critical factor during sustained very high intensity exercise.

Walker (1979) provides a succinct summary of the creatine phosphate shuttle as follows:

The picture that emerges then, is that PCr and creatine can serve as auxiliary energy messengers between mitochondria and the cytosolic sites of ATP utilization. At the mitochondrial site, newly synthesized ATP enters the intermembrane space, where a portion is utilized by Mi-CK for the formation of PCr. The resulting ADP is then favorably situated for transport by translocase into the mitochondrial matrix in exchange for matrix ATP. The PCr formed, unlike ATP, does not compete with

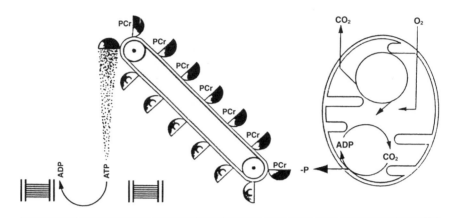

Figure 2.3 A simplified diagram of the phosphocreatine shuttle. Modified from *Podium Kreatin.*

ADP for transport by translocase. In muscle cells, PCr diffuses to the myofibrils, where its small size permits rapid penetration between the myofilaments to reach the CK isozyme located at the M line. There PCr regenerates ATP from the ADP formed during contraction.

> Dietary creatine intake accounts for about half of the body's daily need for creatine, with the remainder obtained through endogenous creatine synthesis from the amino acids glycine, arginine, and methionine.

Adenosine Diphosphate and Hydrogen Ion Buffer; Oxidative Processes

In addition to the role that creatine plays in the phosphagen energy system, it is also intimately involved in metabolic control in several ways (Hochachka 1994; Newsholme and Beis 1996; Saks et al. 1978, 1987; Saks and Ventura-Clapier 1992). First, PCr serves as a cellular buffer through the following reaction:

$$PCr^{2-} + ADP^{3-} + H^+ \rightarrow ATP^{4-} + Cr$$

> Phosphocreatine may serve as a cellular buffer through the following reaction: $PCr^{2-} + ADP^{3-} + H^+ \rightarrow ATP^{4-} + Cr$. It has been proposed that one of the primary functions of the phosphagen system is to buffer elevations in ADP rather than to simply resynthesize ATP—a possible means to prevent premature fatigue.

This buffer is not inconsequential. It has been proposed that one of the primary functions of the phosphagen system is to buffer elevations in ADP rather than to simply resynthesize ATP (Newsholme and Beis 1996). Marked elevations in ADP have been reported to have an inhibitory effect on some ATP reactions. Most cellular ATPases utilize ATP, and therefore rapid accumulation of end-product ADP and adenosine monophosphate (AMP) will significantly alter the equilibrium kinetics around the cellular ATPase, be it myosin ATPase, sarcoplasmic reticulum calcium ATPase, or other regulatory ATPases (Ma et al. 1996), possibly slowing muscle filament cross-bridge cycling (Clark 1997).

As noted in subsequent chapters, some studies with creatine supplementation used plasma ammonia and hypoxanthine as markers of skeletal muscle adenine nucleotide loss. Mujika and Padilla (1997) reported that when the ATP hydrolysis rate within the muscle exceeds the ADP rephosphorylation rate through oxidative processes, anaerobic glycolysis, or PCr breakdown, ATP is resynthesized via the myokinase reaction, resulting in the formation of AMP. Adenosine monophosphate is then deaminated via the adenylate deaminase enzyme in the first reaction of the purine nucleotide cycle, leading to the depletion of the adenine nucleotide pool and the eventual production of ammonia and hypoxanthine.

If the capacity of the creatine phosphate shuttle could be increased, very high intensity exercise performance might be improved. At the sarcomeres, where large amounts of ATP are hydrolyzed, the immediate rephosphorylation of ADP by MM-CK maintains a lower ADP concentration. This prevents inactivation of myosin ATPases and loss of adenine nucleotides (van Deursen et al. 1993).

In addition, PCr may help buffer hydrogen ions (H^+). ATP hydrolysis occurring during muscle contraction, and concurrent function of the calcium and sodium pumps, release protons; conversely, during resynthesis of ATP, protons are taken up (Walker 1979), as illustrated in this reaction:

$$H^+ + PCr + ADP \leftrightarrow Cr + ATP$$

It has been suggested that increases in hydrogen ions (and decreases in pH levels) during intense exercise contribute to fatigue. Consequently, increasing the capacity of cells to buffer H^+ may serve to attenuate the decline in pH levels during intense exercise and may delay fatigue.

PCr may help buffer H^+. Increasing the cell's capacity to buffer H^+ may serve to attenuate the decline in pH levels during intense exercise and may delay fatigue.

Finally, tissue oxygen uptake ($\dot{V}O_2$) has been reported to change in parallel to changes in creatine content (Cerretelli and diPrampero 1987; Mahler 1980; Saks 1996; Whipp and Mahler 1980). It has been hypothesized that CK may serve as a rate-limiting enzyme in tissue oxygen uptake (see figure 2.4). Fluctuations in the concentrations of creatine and PCr may control cellular metabolic activity to a greater degree than alterations in the concentrations of ATP, ADP, and Pi. For example, Ma et al. (1996) present the hypothesis that creatine produced at sites of high metabolic activity, as it diffuses back into the mitochondria to be rephosphorylated to PCr through the action of Mi-CK, may be the respiratory signal to the mitochondria. Proponents of this creatine control theory contend that it provides a viable explanation as to the relationship between oxygen uptake kinetics and alterations in the creatine/PCr ratio. If this is the case, then increasing creatine and PCr through creatine supplementation may have a greater metabolic effect than originally contended.

Some investigators hypothesize that creatine may function as a respiratory signal to the mitochondria, possibly influencing oxygen kinetics during exercise.

Other Functions of Creatine

Energy characteristics of creatine are important for tissues other than skeletal muscle. A small percentage of the body's creatine stores are found in the heart, and CK activities have been found associated with the plasma membrane of heart cells (Walker 1979). Over the last several decades, there has been a significant amount of research on the effects of creatine, PCr, and CK on myocardial metabolism (Conway et al. 1996a, 1996b; Saks 1996; Saks et al. 1996). The reason is that in addition to the important metabolic roles of CK, creatine, and PCr described earlier, reduced creatine availability has been associated with heart failure, ischemia, increased prevalence of ventricular arrhythmias, and instability of myocardial cell membranes during ischemia (Conway et al. 1996a, 1996b; Saks 1996; Saks et al. 1996). Consequently, intravenously administered PCr and oral creatine have been proposed as cardioprotective agents for people with ischemic heart disease; related research findings are discussed in chapter 9.

A small amount of creatine is also found in central and peripheral nervous system tissue. There is evidence that creatine may play an important role in brain function as well as in neuromuscular control. For example, infants born with the inability to endogenously synthesize creatine (i.e., an inborn error in creatine synthesis) experience abnormal mental, neuromuscular, and physical maturation (Stöckler and Hanefeld 1997; Stockler et al. 1994, 1996a, 1996b, 1997). Oral creatine supplementation in infants with inborn errors in creatine synthesis (4 to 8 g/day for up to 25 months) has been found to promote normal mental and physical development. Additionally, oral creatine supplementation has been proposed as a treatment for selected neuromuscular diseases such as mitochondrial cytopathies (Tarnopolsky et al. 1997). An expanded discussion of these topics is presented in chapter 9.

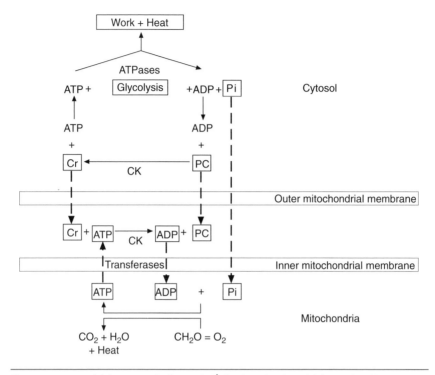

Figure 2.4 Model for control of muscle $\dot{V}O_2$ via mitochondrial creatine kinase (CK). Adapted from Cerretelli and di Prampero (1987) and Mahler (1980).

Creatine plays important roles in heart and nerve tissues, influencing cardiac and neural functions.

Creatine also may be a signal to stimulate protein synthesis, possibly by promoting intracellular fluid retention and cellular osmotic pressure (Bessman and Savabi 1988; Ingwall 1976; Kreider 1998a; Kreider et al. 1998b; Vandenberghe et al. 1997a; Ziegunfuss et al. 1997). In support of this theory, Ingwall (1976) reported that adding creatine to incubated skeletal muscle cells enhanced myosin synthesis in vitro. Chapter 8 presents a fuller discussion of this topic.

Creatine may be a signal to stimulate protein synthesis, possibly by promoting intracellular fluid retention and increasing cellular osmotic pressure.

Catabolism and Excretion

In his extensive review of the scientific literature on creatine, Walker (1979) indicated that other than the energy-related functions of PCr, the only known transformation of PCr in vertebrates is its irreversible nonenzymatic conversion to creatinine. Measurements on rat skeletal muscle in vivo indicate that the cell loses 1.7% to 2.5% of total creatine per day on average. The similarity to the rate of loss of creatine from the cell as creatinine has led to the proposal that creatine efflux from the cell occurs almost exclusively as creatinine (Clark et al. 1996b). Most creatinine is generated in the skeletal muscle, the major storage site of creatine and subsequent creatinine production, and the conversion appears to be spontaneous (Clark 1997; Crim et al., 1975; 1976).

> Other than the energy-related functions of PCr, the only known transformation of PCr is its irreversible nonenzymatic conversion to creatinine. In healthy individuals, approximately 1.6% of the daily creatine pool is degraded to creatinine in the muscle and excreted in the urine.

In healthy individuals, approximately 1.6% of the daily creatine pool is degraded to creatinine in the muscle. Once generated, creatinine enters the circulation by simple diffusion and is filtered in a nonenergy-dependent process by the glomerulus and excreted in urine (Chanutin 1926; Greenhaff 1997b; Walker 1960a, 1960b, 1979). Daily renal excretion of creatinine approximates 2 g, but this amount may vary considerably among individuals depending on total muscle mass. Creatinine levels have been reported to increase mildly in response to intense exercise (Irving et al. 1986, 1990; Janssen et al. 1989; Kargotich et al. 1997; Long et al. 1990). Also, creatinine excretion may increase as much as 10-fold with certain pathological conditions such as kidney disease.

Chapter Summary

Creatine is a naturally occurring amino acid found in the body primarily in muscle tissue. The daily requirement of creatine is about 2 to 3 g/day depending on body size and daily turnover rate. About half of the daily needs are obtained from the diet primarily from meat and fish. Creatine obtained from dietary sources is absorbed intact in the small intestine. The remaining daily need for creatine is synthesized from the amino acids glycine, arginine, and methionine primarily in the liver. The normal creatine content in muscle is about 120-125 mmol/kg dm although dietary availability of creatine may result in lower or higher creatine stores. Creatine supplementation has been reported to increase creatine stores to as much as 160 mmol/kg dm. Most of the creatine in muscle is stored in the form of PCr. Metabolically, PCr serves as an important contributor to energy metabolism during high-intensity exercise. Increasing the availability of PCr would theoretically enhance the ability to maintain power output during intense exercise as well as promote recovery between bouts of intense exercise. However, creatine also serves to buffer acidity, plays an important role in many creatine kinase reactions, is intimately involved in the creatine phosphate shuttle, and may help regulate oxidative metabolism.

Consequently, the availability of creatine and PCr may also affect exercise bouts involving the glycolytic and oxidative energy systems. A small amount of creatine is stored in the heart and brain and is intimately involved in myocardial metabolism as well as brain and neural function. Finally, creatine has been reported to stimulate protein synthesis. Therefore, increasing the availability of creatine and PCr may affect metabolism in a variety of ways. The normal daily turnover rate of creatine (2-3 g) is about 1.6% of the creatine pool. Creatine is degraded primarily in muscle to creatinine and excreted as creatinine in urine.

3

Creatine Supplementation: Theory, Protocols, and Effects

Scientists have investigated the effect of various nutritional supplements or dietary strategies on exercise or sport performance for over a century, and have discovered several that may provide an ergogenic effect to some athletes under specific conditions. For example, the muscles of aerobic endurance athletes are generally rich in oxidative muscle fibers (type I red and type II red)—fibers that store substantial amounts of glycogen. Glycogen is derived from dietary carbohydrate. When it was discovered that muscle glycogen is the major energy substrate for high-intensity aerobic endurance exercise, such as marathon running, scientists experimented with various carbohydrate-feeding techniques in attempts to increase muscle glycogen stores. Today, most marathoners practice carbohydrate-supplementation strategies, known popularly as carbohydrate loading, during the week preceding the race.

Athletes in high-power anaerobic sports, such as sprinters, generally have an abundance of type II white muscle fibers—fibers that are rich in phosphocreatine (PCr) (Boicelli et al. 1989; Greenhaff et al. 1992; Harris et al. 1992). These type II fibers are designed to produce very high intensity anaerobic power. In the early 1990s, research associates from England and Sweden, namely Paul Greenhaff, Roger Harris, and Eric Hultman, initiated contemporary research to investigate the ergogenic potential of creatine supplementation, using a technique somewhat analogous to carbohydrate loading.

Athletes in high-power, anaerobic sports, such as sprinters, generally have an abundance of type II white muscle fibers, fibers that are rich in PCr.

Conway and Clark (1996b) rank PCr with carbohydrate, fat, and protein and other compounds as central components of the metabolic system involved in the provision of energy for work and exercise performance. The purpose of this chapter is to review the theoretical basis underlying creatine supplementation, various supplementation protocols, and the effects of supplementation on body stores of total creatine (TCr), including free creatine (FCr) and PCr.

Human Energy and Fatigue

In a recent review, Sahlin (1998) notes that although our knowledge of the mechanism and the limits of the muscle contraction process has been extended considerably during recent years, the mechanism(s) of fatigue is still not fully understood. The cause of exercise-induced fatigue is dependent on the intensity and duration of the exercise task, and central (central nervous system) or peripheral (skeletal muscle) fatigue may be related to numerous factors, including increased formation of depressant neurotransmitters, decreased levels of metabolic substrates, impaired metabolic processes, disturbed acid-base balance, decreased oxygen transport, disturbed electrolyte balance, and increased core body temperature resulting in hyperthermia.

Although the mechanisms of fatigue are still not fully understood, the classic hypothesis suggests that muscle fatigue is caused by failure of the energetic processes to generate ATP at a sufficient rate.

Sahlin (1998) has reviewed the classic hypothesis that muscle fatigue is caused by failure of the energetic processes to generate adenosine triphosphate (ATP) at a sufficient rate. For example, relative to aerobic endurance performance, as supportive evidence for this hypothesis Sahlin cites findings that interventions increasing the power (i.e., aerobic training) or capacity (i.e., carbohydrate loading) of the energetic processes result in enhanced performance and a delayed onset of fatigue. Similarly, factors that impair the energetic processes (i.e., depletion of muscle glycogen) have a negative influence on performance.

Relative to very high intensity anaerobic exercise, resistance or strength training likewise enhances performance and delays fatigue. Substrate availability for anaerobic exercise may also influence fatigue processes. Wilson (1994) indicates that in muscle cells, the concentration of high-energy phosphate bonds is approximated by the concentration of ATP plus that of PCr, noting that this sum is small compared to the amount of ATP utilization during a few seconds of mild exercise. Wilson also notes that compared to ATP, skeletal muscle has somewhat higher reserves of phosphocreatine, but that these are still too small to sustain more than a few contractions of the muscle.

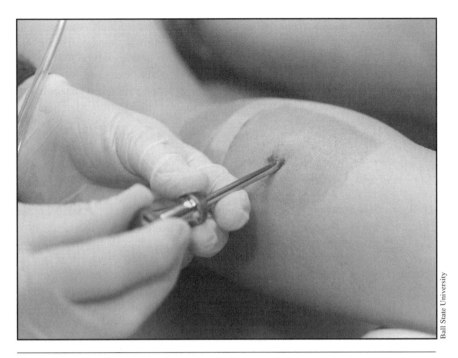

Ball State University

Figure 3.1 Muscle biopsies have shown that sprinters have high concentrations of phosphocreatine (PCr).

Sahlin (1998) states that the amount of energy that can be produced from PCr is rather small and is limited by the intramuscular store, noting that the muscle content of PCr is about 15% higher in fast-twitch fibers than in slow-twitch fibers. Research has shown that very high intensity anaerobic exercise may lead to significant decrements in muscle PCr concentration (Miller et al. 1987, 1988; Tesch et al. 1986). In this regard, Hultman and Greenhaff (1991) indicated that during short-lasting near-maximal exercise (0-30 sec), the anaerobic utilization of muscle PCr and glycogen will fuel muscle contraction; evidence is available to indicate that fatigue during this type of exercise is related to the inability of type II fibers to maintain the very high rate of ATP resynthesis required. It has been suggested that this results from a rapid depletion of type II fiber PCr stores and an insufficiency of the glycogenolytic rate to compensate for the fall in ATP production when the PCr store is depleted. In this situation the force generation has to decrease because of insufficient energy supplies.

During short-lasting, very high intensity exercise (0-30 sec), the anaerobic utilization of muscle PCr is a major factor fueling muscle contraction.

In research addressing energy metabolism in single muscle fibers during maximal sprint exercise, Greenhaff et al. (1992) reported an almost total depletion of PCr in type II fibers, and those subjects with the highest preexercise type II fiber PCr content had the smallest decline in power output during exercise. Similarly to benefits of carbohydrate supplementation for aerobic endurance performance (Hawley et al., 1997), could creatine supplementation enhance very high intensity anaerobic performance?

Theoretical Ergogenic Benefits

The theoretical ergogenic benefits of creatine supplementation are related to the role of creatine and PCr in muscle energetics, as discussed in chapter 2. Although creatine supplementation may, theoretically, be ergogenic for very high intensity, short-term exercise performance dependent upon the ATP-PCr energy system, it may also theoretically benefit performance in less intense, longer-duration exercise bouts.

Several pioneers investigating the ergogenic effects of creatine supplementation, along with their colleagues (Harris et al. 1992; Hultman et al. 1996), have proposed several mechanisms whereby creatine supplementation could be ergogenic for very-high-intensity and high-intensity exercise. These mechanisms involve (1) increased resting levels of PCr availability to serve as an immediate buffer to ATP use during exercise; (2) increased resting levels of free creatine (FCr) to increase the PCr resynthesis rate during and after exercise, facilitating energy translocation from the mitochondria to sites of ATP utilization; and (3) enhanced buffering of hydrogen ions (H^+) to reduce excess acidity in the muscle cell. Other ergogenic mechanisms may also be operative.

Phosphocreatine Availability

Intramuscular supplies of both high-energy phosphagens ATP and PCr are limited; it is estimated that the combined total sustains high-intensity exercise for approximately 10 sec in very-high-intensity exercise (Balsom et al. 1994). Sahlin (1998) notes that the breakdown of PCr is the energetic process that can sustain the highest rate of ATP production. The maximum rate of PCr breakdown observed in vivo is close to the maximal in vitro rate of ATP hydrolysis by the contractile protein. Therefore, it seems plausible that the release of energy during very short bursts of activity (e.g., the high jump, shot put, and the start of a 100 m sprint) is not limited by the rate of ATP generation through PCr breakdown but rather by intrinsic limitations of the contractile proteins or by motor unit recruitment.

However, Sahlin (1998) also points out that on the basis of thermodynamic considerations, one would expect the maximum rate of PCr breakdown to decrease when the PCr content of the muscle decreases. Availability of PCr may therefore be a limiting factor on power output even before the muscle content of PCr is totally depleted. This may explain why the running speed at the end of a 100 m race decreases despite the fact that PCr is not completely depleted. Other researchers (Greenhaff 1997b; Hirvonen et al. 1987; Hultman et al. 1991) also conclude that PCr availability is generally accepted as one factor limiting exercise capacity during short-term supramaximal exercise. Muscle PCr concentrations also were reported to decrease by 86-99% in more prolonged (approximately 50 sec) exercise tasks to fatigue (Katz et al., 1986).

Theoretically, then, creatine supplementation could increase [TCr], possibly facilitating the generation of intramuscular [PCr] and subsequent ATP formation principally in fast-twitch muscle fibers, prolonging the duration of high-intensity physical activity (Balsom et al. 1994; Casey et al. 1996). Some findings (Casey et al. 1996; Greenhaff et al. 1994b) suggest that oral creatine supplementation attenuates ATP degradation during intense muscle contraction, by as much as 30%, probably by better maintaining the rate of ATP resynthesis from adenosine diphosphate (ADP).

As Sahlin (1998) acknowledges, some scientists argue that since muscle ATP remains practically unchanged during exhaustive exercise, it is unlikely that fatigue is caused by energy deficiency. However, Sahlin suggests that this line of reasoning may be too simplistic, since temporal and spatial gradients of adenine nucleotides may exist in contracting muscle. Furthermore, the link between energy deficiency and fatigue may be related to increases in the products of ATP hydrolysis (i.e., ADP, adenosine monophosphate [AMP], or inorganic phosphate [Pi]) rather than decreases in ATP per se. A small decrease in ATP will cause relatively large increases in ADP and AMP because of the lower concentrations of these latter compounds. As pointed out by Sahlin, recent studies have shown that under a variety of conditions, muscle fatigue is associated with increased catabolism of adenine nucleotides to inosine monophosphate (IMP) and ammonia, supporting the hypothesis that in many cases, fatigue is related to a mismatch between utilization and generation of ATP.

In this regard, PCr acts as a temporal buffer of cytosolic ADP accumulation during exercise (Casey et al. 1996). The accumulation of IMP, ammonia, or hypoxanthine after high-intensity exercise is an indication of adenine nucleotide degradation, so evidence of lower postexercise levels of these substances after creatine supplementation may suggest an enhanced rate of ATP formation from ADP. Mujika and Padilla (1997) believe that an increased muscle PCr concentration achieved through supplementary creatine ingestion would most likely induce an enhanced rephosphorylation of ADP during muscular exercise, which would result in a lesser adenine nucleotide degradation, or preservation of ATP. This suggestion is supported by studies showing that the accumulation of plasma ammonia and hypoxanthine is reduced during maximal exercise following creatine ingestion (Greenhaff 1997b).

Increased Phosphocreatine Resynthesis

Bogdanis et al. (1995) reported that PCr resynthesis during the recovery period from high-intensity exercise appears to be a determining factor in restoration of energy for a subsequent high-intensity exercise task. In this regard, Greenhaff (1995) indicated that the availability of FCr has been ascribed a central role in the control of PCr resynthesis, and he also noted (1997b) that the acceleration of postexercise PCr resynthesis would be expected to increase muscle contractile capability by maintaining ATP turnover during exercise. For this reason, creatine supplementation might be recommended for some athletes such as sprinters, as some evidence suggests that they experience slower resynthesis of muscle PCr after exercise designed to deplete muscle [PCr] by 50-60%—at least as compared to endurance athletes who have higher rates of oxidative metabolism (McCully et al. 1992).

Clark (1996) noted that the rapid resynthesis of PCr is likely to be oxidative in origin, and raised the question: Do increased PCr and creatine cause an increase in oxidative phosphorylation? Because of the presence of a specific creatine kinase (CK) isoenzyme within the mitochondria, it appears very likely that the added creatine will increase PCr resynthesis. Clark indicates that this is so because mitochondrial creatine kinase (Mi-CK) is found on the outer surface of the inner mitochondrial membrane and is functionally coupled to oxidative phosphorylation. Thus, the Mi-CK system stimulates mitochondrial respiration because of elevated intermembrane space [ADP].

Chapter 5 details the effect of creatine supplementation on PCr resynthesis and actual exercise or sport performance dependent upon the ATP-PCr (phosphagen) energy system.

Reduced Muscle Acidity

Walker (1979) indicates that glycolysis may be modulated by PCr. Phosphofruc-tokinase, a major regulatory glycolytic enzyme, may be partially inhibited by PCr working in concert with inhibitory ATP. During strenuous muscular activity, this inhibition would be relieved by a decrease in PCr levels and increase in Pi concentration, and glycolysis would increase. Anaerobic glycolysis increases lactic acid accumulation, with increased hydrogen ion (H^+) concentration a possible contributor to muscle fatigue.

Phosphocreatine acts as the principal metabolic buffer in muscle, accounting for approximately 30% of the total muscle buffer capacity (Hultman and Sahlin 1980). Adenosine triphosphate resynthesis from ADP and PCr consumes a H^+ in the process, so utilization of PCr will contribute to the buffering of H^+ (Harris et al. 1992). Rossiter et al. (1996) suggest that one benefit of an elevated buffer value is that it should allow the muscle to accumulate more lactic acid before reaching a limiting muscle pH, and thus allow more high-intensity exercise to be performed. Blood lactate levels, if lowered, might be indicative of less reliance on anaerobic glycolysis for a standardized exercise bout.

Although some researchers report lower postexercise lactic acid levels following creatine supplementation, even in spite of a higher workload (Söderlund et al. 1994), most studies reveal no effect of creatine supplementation on blood lactate levels (Birch et al., 1994; Burke et al., 1996; Dawson et al., 1995; Green et al. 1993;

Greenhaff et al. 1993b; Maughan 1995; Mujika et al. 1996; Peyrebrune et al., 1998). However, if greater work output is achieved with creatine supplementation, the lack of significant differences in lactate could be interpreted as less reliance on anaerobic glycolysis.

In chapter 6 we will detail the effect of creatine supplementation on actual exercise or sport performance dependent upon anaerobic glycolysis.

Oxidative Metabolism

Although PCr breakdown to provide ATP is an anaerobic process, several investigators speculate that creatine supplementation, possibly by increasing PCr, may modify substrate utilization and possibly improve performance during prolonged, submaximal exercise (Stroud et al. 1994). Using an animal model, Brannon et al. (1997) reported that creatine supplementation, in combination with training, increased the level of citrate synthase (CS) activity, a marker of oxidative capacity, in both fast- and slow-twitch muscle. In the soleus, creatine supplementation alone caused an increase in CS activity that matched the gains resulting from training. The combination of training and supplementation did not cause any further increases in CS activity in this muscle. In the plantaris, however, supplementation alone had no effect on CS activity, while training caused an increase, and the combination of training and supplementation had an additive effect. However, these investigators had no explanation for these effects of creatine supplementation. This effect may possibly be attributed to the role of creatine in the transport of ATP between the cytosol and mitochondria, as discussed in chapter 2.

Bangsbo et al. (1990) suggested that PCr contributes significantly to ATP resynthesis during longer constant-work exercise bouts, indicating that in an exercise task with a mean performance time of 3.2 min, the alactic contribution from PCr was approximately 15-20% of the total anaerobic energy demand. The muscle PCr stores decreased by 60%, approximating the value reported for 11-30 sec of all-out sprinting. These investigators noted that because PCr may aid ATP resynthesis for up to 3 min, albeit in a decreasing role with time and intensity of work, and because of the potential for PCr to act as an energy shuttle between the mitochondria and myofibril, creatine supplementation may possibly be an ergogenic aid during longer anaerobic work bouts. Although there is a strong anaerobic component to an exercise task of 3 min duration, there also is a significant aerobic component.

Engelhardt et al. (1998) note that aerobic endurance athletes have to use anaerobic work only to a certain extent but that this type of work may influence their performance in certain situations—such as anaerobic energy expenditure during intermittent and finishing spurts. For example, removal of the drafting rule in international triathlons changes the character of the competition and requires intermittent anaerobic work within an aerobic endurance exercise task on a high-intensity level. Also, Bangsbo (1994) noted that although aerobic energy production appears to account for more than 90% of total energy consumption in soccer games, anaerobic energy production nevertheless plays an essential role. He observes that during intensive exercise periods within a game, PCr, and to a lesser extent the stored ATP, are utilized. Both compounds are partly restored during a subsequent prolonged rest period. In such cases, PCr resynthesis during less intense exercise periods, as discussed earlier, may be augmented by creatine supplementation.

Chapter 7 provides further detail on the effect of creatine supplementation on actual exercise or sport performance dependent upon aerobic glycolysis, or oxidative metabolism.

Enhanced Training

Several investigators have suggested that creatine supplementation could benefit athletes over the long term by enabling a higher training load, improving repetitive-interval sprint capacity, reducing training fatigue, and possibly accelerating muscle hypertrophy (Greenhaff 1997a; Vandenberghe et al. 1997a; Viru et al. 1994; Volek et al., 1999).

Increased Body Mass

Increased body mass, preferably increased fat-free body weight, or muscle mass, might be advantageous in sports requiring a high absolute power output to overcome an external object or to resist, for instance, the inertia of another body (Fogelholm and Saris 1998).

Creatine supplementation may influence body mass, and body composition with respect to such factors as increased fat-free body mass or muscle mass, in several ways. Volek et al. (1997b) note that creatine is an osmotically active substance; thus an increase in intracellular creatine concentration may likely induce influx of water into the cell. An increased body water content would increase body mass. However, Volek and his colleagues (1997b) also indicate that an increase in intramuscular cell water may be seen as an anabolic proliferative signal. Citing supportive research by Häussinger et al. (1993), Volek and colleagues speculate that an increased cellular hydration induced by creatine supplementation may increase protein synthesis, decrease protein degradation, and thus increase fat-free mass. In his review, Clark (1997) suggests that elevation of PCr in the muscle cell is also capable of stimulating protein synthesis, somewhat similar to that induced by exercise or insulin as suggested by Bessman and Mohan (1992). However, acute creatine supplementation does not appear to influence several hormones, such as testosterone and cortisol, that might influence body mass (Volek et al. 1997b).

In an excellent review regarding the effect of creatine supplementation on body composition, Volek and Kraemer (1996) noted that creatine may be the chemical signal coupling increased muscular activity to increased contractile protein synthesis in hypertrophy. Summarizing key investigations by Ingwall (1976) and his colleagues (Ingwall et al. 1972, 1974), who studied the effects of creatine on mononucleated muscle cells isolated from breast muscle in chick embryos, Volek and Kraemer (1996) made the following observations from these animal models:

1. Creatine supplied in vitro increases the rate of synthesis of myosin heavy chain and actin formed both in vitro and in vivo.
2. Creatine affects only the rate of synthesis, not the rate of degradation.
3. Creatine affects only cells already synthesizing muscle proteins, not the cellular events during myoblast proliferation or during cell fusion.
4. Creatine increases overall synthesis of ribonucleic acid (RNA) and seems to preferentially induce specific classes of RNA.
5. The effect of creatine is manifested in different stages of the synthesis of muscle proteins; however, the primary effect is connected with the nucleus and is accomplished at the transcription level.

However, also discussing Ingwall's work, Walker (1979) indicated that the relevance of this research approach to hypertrophy of adult muscle is not yet clear in view of the relatively high level of endogenous creatine already present in adult muscle cells; the modulating effect of creatine might therefore already be maximal in adult muscle.

The effect of creatine supplementation on body mass and body composition is detailed in chapter 8.

How Creatine Supplementation Prevents Fatigue

Theoretically, creatine supplementation may help prevent fatigue by one or more of the following mechanisms:

a. Increasing PCr availability
   A higher initial muscle PCr concentration may help sustain muscle contraction.

b. Increasing PCr resynthesis
   A higher initial level of FCr may help resynthesize more PCr during recovery.

c. Reducing muscle acidity
   Phosphocreatine acts as the principal metabolic buffer in muscle, consuming a H^+ in the process of resynthesizing ATP from ADP. An elevated buffer value may allow the muscle to accumulate more lactic acid before reaching a limiting muscle pH, thus increasing the duration of high-intensity exercise.

d. Enhancing various facets of oxidative metabolism
   In combination with training, creatine may increase the level of citrate synthase activity, a marker of oxidative capacity. Also, some endurance athletes may use PCr during intensive exercise periods within an athletic contest and may benefit from enhanced PCr resynthesis during aerobic recovery periods.

e. Enhancing training
   Increased creatine or PCr may enable athletes to reach a higher training load, improve repetitive-interval sprint capacity, reduce training fatigue, and possibly accelerate muscle hypertrophy—all factors that may enhance competitive performance.

f. Increasing body mass
   An increased fat-free body weight, or muscle mass, might be advantageous in sports requiring a high absolute power output to resist the inertia of another body or to overcome an external object.

Theoretical Ergolytic Effects

Although creatine supplementation may possibly be ergogenic for certain exercise or sport endeavors, some suggest that it may also be ergolytic—may impair performance—in other types of events. Clark (1996) cautioned that the apparent increase in anaerobic metabolism caused by creatine supplementation may produce more lactate and therefore make an athlete more prone to lactic acidosis.

A creatine supplementation-induced increase in body mass, particularly if not muscle mass, could be detrimental to performance in sports in which the body mass needs to be moved efficiently from one point to another. For example, an increased body mass could be detrimental to distance runners, as they would have to expend more oxidative energy to move the extra mass. However, for sprinters, theoretical increases in power production could counterbalance the potential adverse effects of an increased body mass. Relative to this latter point, a similar situation exists with marathon runners; they gain body mass with carbohydrate loading, but the more efficient carbohydrate energy source appears to counterbalance this effect and leads to performance enhancement.

Theoretically, creatine supplementation may impair exercise or sport performance by increasing body mass; this may decrease metabolic efficiency in tasks in which the body mass needs to be moved efficiently from one point to another.

The ergolytic effects of creatine supplementation will be discussed in various contexts in chapters 5 through 7.

Sport Performance Implications

On the basis of these theoretical considerations, creatine supplementation may benefit performance in a variety of exercise or sport endeavors. Increased PCr availability could improve sprint performance, such as in the 100 m and 200 m dash in track. Increased PCr resynthesis could benefit performance in repetitive, high-intensity exercise tasks with frequent rest intervals, including those in individual and team sports such as tennis and ice hockey. A theoretical model is presented in figure 3.2. Reduced muscle acidity could aid performance in longer anaerobic exercise tasks, such as the 400 m and 800 m run in track. An enhanced training ability could favorably impact performance in a wide variety of sports. An increased body mass, increased muscle mass, and associated gains in strength and power may significantly enhance performance in sports such as competitive weight lifting and American football. Other examples are presented in table 3.1.

Theoretically, creatine supplementation may benefit performance in a variety of exercise or sport endeavors such as very-high-intensity sprint performance; repetitive, high-intensity exercise tasks with frequent rest intervals; longer anaerobic exercise tasks; and resistance-type sport tasks dependent on increased body mass, increased muscle mass, and associated gains in strength and power.

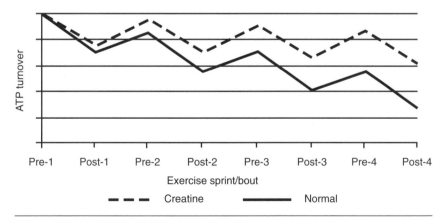

Figure 3.2 Theoretical effect of creatine supplementation on repeated bouts of high-intensity exercise.

Reprinted, by permission, from R. Kreider, 1998, "Creatine supplementation: Analysis of ergogenic value, medical safety and concerns," *JEP Online* 1(1).

Table 3.1 Examples of Sport Performance Theoretically Enhanced by Creatine Supplementation.

Increased PCr

    Track sprints: 100, 200 m

    Swim sprints: 50 m

    Pursuit cycling

Increased PCr resynthesis

    Basketball

    Field hockey

    Football (American)

    Ice hockey

    Lacrosse

    Volleyball

Reduced muscle acidosis

    Downhill skiing

    Rowing

    Swim events: 100, 200 m

    Track events: 400, 800 m

Oxidative metabolism

    Basketball

    Soccer

    Team handball

    Tennis

    Volleyball

Enhanced training

    Most sports

Increased body mass/muscle mass

    Football (American, Australian)

    Bodybuilding

    Heavyweight wrestling

    Power lifting

    Rugby

    Track/field events (Shot put; javelin; discus)

    Weightlifting

Forms of Creatine

Creatine is found naturally in foods, particularly in meat. For early research with creatine supplementation, the creatine was extracted from animal flesh—an expensive process. Today, commercial creatine supplements are produced through chemical synthesis in North America, Asia, and Europe.

Although creatine synthesis is a proprietary process among manufacturers, it is quite common to use another muscle-related compound, sarcosine (or sarcosinate salts), as the principal starting material for the commercial synthesis of creatine. As with creatine synthesis, the starting material used is also synthetically produced. Sarcosine is a component of human metabolism; chemically it is N-methylglycine (a relative of glycine, one of the precursor amino acids in the body's production of creatine). The synthetic chemical cyanamide is also used as a primary starting material. Organic solvent-water mixtures are used as the reaction medium. The purification process removes any residual amounts of reaction components and intermediates.

Creatine monohydrate is the most commonly available creatine supplement and the form primarily used in most research studies. However, other forms are available. Creatine phosphate is sold in small quantities. It is an extremely expensive form of creatine, which likely curtails its widespread distribution and use. Any effect of creatine phosphate ingested orally would be mediated by creatine alone, since gut phosphatase enzymes would readily cleave off the phosphate portion of the molecule, liberating FCr. Additionally, serum possesses high phosphatase activity, leading to rapid breakdown of intravenously administered creatine phosphate to creatine and phosphate (Saks and Strumia 1993). Limited data suggest that PCr infusions may enhance physical training intensity (Clark 1996), and only a few published studies have used oral creatine phosphate to evaluate its effects on exercise performance or health. Creatine phosphate is used in various countries as an injectable drug primarily for medical reasons. However, as Clark (1996) notes, the use of intravenous PCr must be undertaken only under the guidance of a qualified physician.

Creatine monohydrate is the most commonly available creatine supplement and the form primarily used in most research studies. However, other forms of creatine are available, such as creatine citrate and creatine phosphate

---

Creatine citrate is another form of creatine sold as a supplement; here too there appear to be no published studies showing differences in absorption, muscle creatine retention, or functional parameters such as changes in muscle performance or body composition.

Commercial creatine supplements are available in a variety of forms, including powder, tablets, gel, liquid, chewing gum, and candy. Some commercial products blend creatine monohydrate with other substances such as carbohydrate, proteins, vitamins and minerals, amino acids, and even herbal extracts and phytochemicals.

Commercial creatine supplements are available in a variety of forms, including powder, tablets, gel, liquid, chewing gum, and candy. Micronized creatine, designed to dissolve better in fluid, leave less residue in the cup, and enhance intestinal absorption, is also available. Because some studies have indicated that glucose, sodium, and taurine may enhance creatine uptake by the muscle cell (Kreider et al. 1997b), some commercial products blend creatine monohydrate with other substances. For example, Phosphagain™ contains carbohydrate, protein, fat, creatine, taurine, yeast-derived RNA, and L-glutamine. Other commercial products contain dietary proteins, vitamins, and minerals, other amino acids and biochemicals, and even herbal extracts and phytochemicals.

Quality control ensuring the purity of creatine monohydrate employs various analytical chemistry techniques, including high-performance liquid chromatography (HPLC), high-performance capillary electrophoresis (HPCE), fluorescence detection, and various "wet" chemical quantification methods. Creatine monohydrate intended for use as a dietary supplement should be subjected to analytical methods characterized by high specificity and sensitivity (HPLC and HPCE) for each production run.

Dietary supplements containing creatine should list the ingredients on the label, along with recommended daily dosages. Hopefully this listing may provide the buyer with accurate information relative to the actual contents in the supplement, as is not always the case in the dietary supplement industry. Although the implementation of quality control and assurance in production of creatine (or any other dietary supplement) is not mandated by any state or federal regulatory agency (Food and Drug Administration, for example) in North America, most companies appear to require some form of validation of purity from primary creatine manufacturers and suppliers. In choosing a creatine-containing dietary supplement, it is advisable that the prospective buyer request from the distributor independent laboratory analysis records for more than one recent lot of material sold. This request can be made with any distributor of creatine supplements. Plisk and Kreider (1999) have recommended one request the following to obtain quality assurance when purchasing creatine supplements:

1. The product should be manufactured in a USFDA-inspected facility complying with pharmaceutical "Current Good Manufacturing Practices" (the code of federal regulations describing methods, equipment, facilities, and controls used for manufacturing, processing, packing, or holding drugs and foods). This also means that it should comply with "Manufacturing Practices for Nutritional Supplements."

2. A manufacturer's (not distributor's or importer's) certificate of analysis should be provided for random samples from the same batch/lot number on the containers being purchased. Different laboratories may not test for each physical constant listed below, and typical values may vary slightly (hence none are indicated here). However, the vendor takes a big step toward establishing credibility simply by providing this type of documentation:

   - appearance (white to pale cream solid)
   - assay (determined with HPCE or HPLC methods)
   - bulk density
   - mesh size
   - microbiological/pathogenic contamination (e.g., coliforms, e. coli, salmonella, aureus, yeasts/molds) and plate count
   - poisons (e.g., arsenic) and heavy metals (e.g., lead, mercury)

- residual moisture/loss on drying
- residue on ignition (for inorganic materials)

Reputable manufacturers who adhere to these industry standards typically do not hesitate to share this information with potential distributors or vendors.

Dietary supplements containing creatine should list the ingredients on the label, along with recommended daily dosages. Quality-control information should be obtainable from the manufacturer.

Supplementation Protocols

The typical meat-eating individual consumes about 1 g of creatine daily. As the creatine concentration in natural foods is relatively low (approximately 3-5 g of creatine per kilogram of meat or fish) and the process of cooking meat or fish may diminish creatine bioavailability, natural dietary sources may not be a practical means to obtain significant amounts of creatine, particularly the amounts recommended during the creatine-loading phase. Creatine-supplementation protocols involve a loading and a maintenance phase. Various creatine-supplementation strategies have been used in attempts to increase total muscle creatine content, particularly PCr; the results of these are discussed in the next section.

The most commonly used research protocol for creatine loading is to ingest a daily total of 20-30 g of creatine, usually creatine monohydrate, in four equal doses of 5-7 g dissolved in about 250 ml of fluid, over the course of the day (usually early morning, noon, afternoon, and evening) for a period of 5 to 7 days. For those individuals who may be uncomfortable consuming large daily amounts of creatine, Hultman et al. (1996) recommended a lower dose (3 g/day) over a longer time frame (about 1 month) as an alterative creatine-loading protocol. If powder is used, some investigators recommend warm or hot fluids for better dissolution of creatine. Harris et al. (1992) used this technique and reported no detectable formation of creatinine in the fluid.

The most commonly used creatine-loading protocol is to ingest a daily total of 20-30 g of creatine, usually creatine monohydrate, in four equal doses of 5-7 g dissolved in about 250 ml of fluid, over the course of the day—typically early morning, noon, afternoon, and evening—for a period of 5 to 7 days. Based on body weight, the recommended loading dose is 0.3 g/kg body mass per day for a period of 5 to 6 days.

A more prolonged loading protocol, 3 g/day for 28 days, is just as effective as the short-term loading protocol.

Most creatine-loading studies have used absolute doses of creatine, not basing the amount supplemented on body weight. However, Hultman et al. (1996) recommend a loading dose of 0.3 g/kg body mass per day for a period of 5 to 6 days; for a 70 kg individual, this recommended dosage would amount to 21 g/day. Because creatine appears to accumulate primarily in the muscle tissue, some investigators have based creatine supplementation dosages on fat-free mass, or lean body mass.

Following the creatine-loading phase, recommended maintenance dosages are considerably lower. Most research studies have used dosages ranging from 2 to 5 g of creatine per day during the maintenance phase, but a few studies have used higher levels, from 10 to 20 g, for periods ranging from 4 to 10 weeks. Hultman et al. (1996) recommend a maintenance dose of 0.03 g/kg body mass per day; for a 70 kg individual, this recommended dosage would amount to about 2 g/day.

After the creatine-loading phase, recommended maintenance dosages are considerably lower, approximating 2-5 g of creatine per day or 0.03 g/kg body mass per day.

In vitro isolated rat muscle studies have demonstrated that insulin can stimulate muscle creatine transport (Haughland and Chang 1975), so some investigators have theorized that concomitant consumption of simple carbohydrates such as glucose could be an effective complement to creatine supplementation. Green et al. (1996a, 1996b) used 95 g of glucose with each 5 g dose of creatine monohydrate during the loading phase.

Effects of Supplementation

Theoretically, for oral creatine supplementation to be an effective ergogenic, the creatine must be effectively absorbed through the intestines, must increase plasma levels, and must be transported into the muscle cells to increase TCr or PCr above the normal levels needed for energy production or energy substrate resynthesis. In this section we look at some of the effects of creatine supplementation, including various loading and maintenance strategies, and the effects of cessation of supplementation.

Intestinal Absorption and Plasma Levels

As noted in chapter 2, oral creatine supplements appear to be totally absorbed into the body via the intestinal tract, as there are no indications of increased fecal creatine content following supplementation. Although Greenhaff (1997b) has recommended mixing oral creatine powder in a warm liquid because this has been shown to facilitate dissolving of the creatine, most studies have not used hot fluid solutions. Citing his own unpublished work, Greenhaff indicated that creatine when ingested in solution is more effective at raising the plasma creatine concentration than when ingested in tablet form, presumably because intestinal creatine absorption is more rapid when creatine is ingested in solution. However, Vukovich and Michaelis (1999) reported no differences between candy and powder creatine forms. Additionally, micronized creatine has been suggested to increase intestinal absorption of creatine, but no studies have been uncovered to support this suggestion. Almost all ingested creatine monohydrate powder is absorbed.

In one of the first contemporary studies with creatine supplementation, Harris et al. (1992) reported that low doses (1 g creatine monohydrate or less in water) produced only a modest rise in the plasma creatine concentration, whereas a single 5 g dose resulted in a peak concentrations of 690-1,000 μmol/L; in a subset of three subjects with body weights ranging from 76 to 87 kg, the mean peak after 1 hr was 795 μmol/L. Repeated dosing with 5 g every 2 hr sustained the plasma concentration at around 1,000 μmol/L. Greenhaff (1997a) indicated that a 5 g supplement will increase plasma creatine concentration sufficiently over the time course of 1 hr to stimulate muscle creatine uptake, as documented in an animal isolated muscle preparation.

After ingestion of 5 g of creatine, creatine levels in the blood peak during the first hour and then begin to dissipate during the next several hours (Green et al. 1996b). To help maintain peak plasma levels, the recommendation is to ingest creatine in 5 g doses four to five times a day during the loading phase (Harris et al. 1992). Greenhaff also notes that using more than 20 g/day for 5 days provides no additional benefit and is a waste of money.

To help maintain peak creatine plasma levels, the recommendation is to ingest creatine in 5 g doses four to five times a day during the loading phase.

Body Stores and Muscle Concentrations

Several techniques have been utilized to evaluate the effects of oral creatine supplementation on body stores, particularly muscle stores. Direct techniques include muscle biopsy and nuclear magnetic resonance (NMR) or magnetic resonance imaging or spectroscopy, such as ^{31}P-MRS (Kreis et al., 1997). Although direct measurement is the recommended procedure, not all studies addressing the effect of oral creatine supplementation on exercise or sport performance have used direct measurements to determine whether the supplementation protocol actually increases muscle concentrations of TCr and PCr. One indirect technique involves measurement of the urine creatine content, the presumption being that the remainder of the oral supplement was retained in the body. Because some research has shown that oral creatine ingestion may markedly reduce urinary volume during the initial days of creatine supplementation (Hultman et al. 1996), presumably due to increased intracellular water retention, measurement of urine volume has been used as an indirect marker of increased intramuscular creatine content. An increased body mass has also been used as an indirect measure of increased intramuscular creatine concentrations, with the assumption that the increased body mass is associated with the intracellular water increase. However, many studies addressing the effect of creatine supplementation on actual exercise or sport performance used neither direct nor indirect measures of creatine retention.

According to Walker (1979), tissues that undergo the most rapid and drastic changes in energy demand have the highest concentrations of creatine kinase and PCr. Thus creatine, the only guanidine phosphagen found in higher animals, concentrates mostly in skeletal muscle, with lesser amounts in cardiac and smooth muscle, brain, and kidney. Total creatine exists in the muscle as both FCr and PCr. About 60% of the TCr is PCr, and the remainder is FCr. Phosphocreatine concentrations are greatest in fast-twitch, glycolytic white muscle cells, but are somewhat lower in aerobic red skeletal muscle (Walker 1979). The creatine concentration is normally expressed as millimoles per kilogram dry muscle matter or mass (mmol/kg dm).

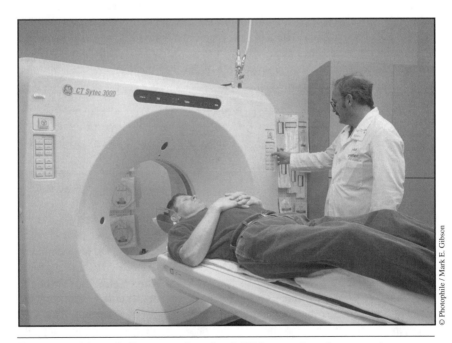

© Photophile / Mark E. Gibson

Figure 3.3 Magnetic Resonance Imaging (MRI) is a noninvasive means to measure muscle creatine concentrations.

In a 70 kg male, normal TCr concentrations approximate 120-125 mmol/kg dm, with 95% in the skeletal muscle (Greenhaff 1995, 1997b). Although vegetarians, when compared to non-vegetarians, have been shown to have lower plasma creatine and creatinine concentrations (Delange et al., 1989), this does not necessarily imply decreased tissue contents; in one study, the two vegetarian subjects had tissue creatine levels within the normal range, 120.0 and 114.6 mmol/kg dm (Harris et al. 1992).

Numerous researchers have reported significant increases in TCr, FCr, and PCr following the most prevalent creatine-loading protocol, one that provides 20-30 g of creatine monohydrate daily for 5 to 6 days. Table 3.2 presents an overview of investigations on the effect of creatine supplementation on muscle creatine and PCr, listing the reference citation, the subject population, the creatine dosage, the method of determination of creatine uptake, and the major findings. The following paragraphs present some of the highlights of these studies.

Using 20-30 g of creatine monohydrate per day for 2 days, Harris et al. (1992) reported a significant increase in the [TCr] of the quadriceps femoris muscle, indicating that 20-40% of the increase in [TCr] was accounted for by [PCr]. However, the authors noted that because of damage inflicted during muscle biopsying it is possible that the increase in situ in PCr content was greater. They also reported that muscle uptake of oral creatine supplementation was greatest in the first two-day supplementation period, accounting for 32% of the dose administered in those subjects receiving the 30 g of creatine monohydrate per day, with smaller increases in subsequent days. No change in ATP content was reported in this study, the values before and after supplementation being 24.9 and 25.8 mmol/kg dm, respectively. Volek et al., (1999) also recently reported no change in ATP, but significant increases in [TCr] (122.9 to 149.9 mmol/kg dm) following 1 week of creatine supplementation (25 g/day); although PCr increased by 22%, this increase was not statistically significant compared to the baseline level. Casey et al. (1996) also reported significant increases in muscle [TCr] (about 18%) and [PCr] (about 10%) after supplementation with 20 g creatine monohydrate for 5 days. Gonzalez de Suso and Prat (1994), using a crossover trial with a 2-week washout period, provided 21 g of creatine monohydrate for 12 days, in three 7 g doses 30 min before meals. The PCr/β-ATP ratio increased 15% in 6 days, and after another 6 days it had increased to 21% of the initial value. Of the 20 subjects who took part in the study, half increased their PCr deposits by more than 15%. Other studies have also shown increases in both [TCr] and [PCr] and the [PCr]/[ATP] ratio (Balsom et al. 1995; Greenhaff et al. 1994b; Hultman et al. 1996; Lemon et al. 1995; Myburgh et al. 1996; Vandenberghe et al. 1996a, 1997a, 1999). During this rapid 5- to 6-day creatine-loading protocol, most of the creatine is absorbed into the muscles in the first few days, and about 30% of the administered dose is absorbed; in subsequent days, only about 15% is absorbed (Greenhaff 1997b). In his review, Greenhaff (1997b) reports that this creatine-loading protocol has been shown to increase muscle TCr concentration by approximately 25 mmol/kg dm in humans.

Table 3.2 Summary of Studies Investigating the Effects of Creatine Supplementation on Muscle Creatine, Phosphocreatine, Adenosine Triphosphate, and Glycogen Concentrations.

Investigator	Year	Population	Creatine dosage grams/day	Method of determination of creatine uptake	Results
Balsom et al.	1995	7 males	20 g/d, 6d	Muscle biopsy	18% increase in resting [TCr] (129 to 152 mmol dry mass). 52% higher [PCr] (70 vs. 46 mmol/kg dry mass) in creatine group following 5 x 6 sec sprints.
Casey et al.	1996	9 males	20 g/d, 5d	Muscle biopsy	[PCr] increased in both type I and II fibers. [TCr] in muscle increased by 23 mmol/kg dry mass. There was 31% less loss in [ATP] despite producing more work in the creatine group. Changes in resting [PCr] in type II fibers were positively correlated to changes in [PCr] during exercise and changes in total work.
Febbraio et al.	1995	6 males	20 g/d, 5d	Muscle biopsy	Significant increases in [TCr] and [PCr] with no effect on [ATP], [ADP], [AMP], or [IMP]. [TCr] stores returned to normal within 28d washout period.
Gordon et al.	1995	17 heart failure patients	20 g/d, 10d	Muscle biopsy	Creatine supplementation significantly increased muscle [TCr] by 17% and [PCr] by 12%.

Green et al.	1996a	21 males	20 g/d, 5d; or 400 g/d of glucose; or creatine + 400 g/d CHO	Muscle biopsy	Creatine ingestion resulted in an 18% increase in [TCr] (122 to 143 mmol/kg dry mass) with no effect on [glycogen] (365 to 366 mmol/kg dry mass). Ingestion of glucose alone resulted in a 4% decrease in [TCr] (130 to 124 mmol/kg dry mass) and a 22% increase in [glycogen] content (338 to 441 mmolkg dry mass). Ingestion of glucose with creatine resulted in a 10% greater increase in [TCr] (124 to 158 mmol/kg dry mass or 27%) and a 48% nonsignificant increase in muscle glycogen (331 to 489 mmol/kg dry mass). Increased muscle [glycogen] was significantly correlated to changes in [TCr].
Greenhaff et al.	1994a	8 males	20 g/d, 5d	Muscle biopsy	Resting [TCr] was increased by 15%. PCr resynthesis was similar at 60 sec recovery but 42% greater following 120 sec recovery after creatine supplementation.
Greenhaff et al.	1993a	10 males 2 females	20 g/d, 5d	Muscle biopsy ^{31}P-MRS	20% increase in [PCr] (55 to 67 mmol/kg dry mass) determined by biopsy. 11% increase in [PCr] (77 to 85 mmol/kg dry mass) determined by ^{31}P-MRS.
Harris et al.	1992	12 males 5 females	20 to 30 g/d taken at 4.5, 7, 10, or 21d	Muscle biopsy	20% increase in [TCr] (127 to 149 mmol/kg dry mass). 36% increase in [PCr] (67 to 91 mmol/kg dry mass). No effect on [ATP].

(continued)

Table 3.2 (continued)

Investigator	Year	Population	Creatine dosage grams/day	Method of determination of creatine uptake	Results
Hultman et al.	1996	31 males	20 g/d, 6d, then 2 g/d, 22d; or, 3 g/d, 28d	Muscle biopsy	Ingesting 20 g/d of creatine for 6d resulted in a 20% increase in [TCr]. Ingesting 2 g/d of creatine thereafter served to maintain muscle [TCr]. [TCr] declined within 30d without ingestion of the 2 g/d maintenance dose. Ingesting 3 g/d of creatine resulted in a gradual increase in muscle [TCr] approaching loading levels in 28d.
Kurosawa et al.	1997	4 males 1 female	30 g/d, 14d	^{31}P-MRS Muscle biopsy	Muscle [creatine] relative to β-ATP levels was increased by 11% in the nontraining and 23% in the trained group.
Lemon	1995	7 males	20 g/d, 5d with 35d washout	^{31}P-MRS	[PCr]/[β-ATP] ratio was increased by 8% (p = 0.10). There was some evidence that the 35d washout was not long enough for [TCr] to return to normal.
Myburgh et al.	1996	13 trained cyclists	20 g/d, 7d; then 2 g/d, 7d	Muscle biopsy	Muscle [TCr] was increased by 21% (121 to 147 mmol/kg dry mass). The increase in [TCr] was significantly correlated to the percentage of type IIb muscle fibers.

Myburgh *(cont.)*

					No significant differences were observed between groups in ATP levels.
Odland et al.	1997	9 males	20 g/d, 3d; with 14d washout	Muscle biopsy	No significant differences were observed between treatments in resting [ATP], [PCr], or [TCr]. The ratio of [TCr]/[ATP] was significantly greater in the creatine-supplemented group.
Rossiter et al.	1996	19 competitive rowers	0.25 g/kg/d, 5d	Urinary [creatine]	Calculated total creatine uptake over the 5d period averaged 35 g with an estimated muscle uptake of 38 mmol/kg dry mass.
Ruden et al.	1996	5 females 4 males	20 g/d, 4d; with 14d washout	Muscle biopsy	Muscle [TCr] was significantly increased by 20 to 21 mmol/kg dry mass. No significant differences were observed between groups in gains in [PCr] (creatine 6.4 vs. placebo 2.5 mmol/kg dry mass).
Thompson et al.	1996	10 female swimmers	2 g/d, 42d	^{31}P-MRS	No significant differences were observed between groups in resting, exercise, or postexercise bioenergetics.
Vandenberghe et al.	1996a	9 males	0.5 g/kg/d or 0.5 g/kg/d with 5 mg/kg/d caffeine, 6d	^{31}P-NMR	No effect on [ATP]. Muscle [PCr] was significantly increased by 4% and 6% in both groups receiving creatine.
Vandenberghe et al.	1997a	19 untrained females	20 g/d, 4d; then 5 g/d, 66d	^{31}P-NMR	NMR-determined total PCr and the ratio of [PCr/[β-ATP] were significantly increased by 6%. These values were maintained during the low-dose supplementation phase.

(continued)

Table 3.2 *(continued)*

Investigator	Year	Population	Creatine dosage grams/day	Method of determination of creatine uptake	Results
Vandenberghe et al.	1999	9 healthy males	25 g/d, 5d	P-NMR	Compared with placebo, 2 and 5 days of creatine supplementation increased resting muscle [PCr] by 11% and 16% respectively.
Volek et al.	1999	19 males	25 g/d, 7d; then 5 g/d, 77d	Muscle biopsy	Muscle [TCr] increased by 22% (122.9 mmol/kg dm to 149.9 mmol/kg dm). Slight drop to 135.9 mmol/L after 12 wk, but still significantly higher than placebo.
Zehnder et al.	1998	8 males 1 female	21 g/d, 5d	^{31}P-MRS	Muscle [PCr] increased by 21% (21.1 to 24.5 mmol/kg dm). Muscle [ATP] increased by 9% (5.6 to 6.1 mmol/kg dm).

Hultman et al. (1996) also reported that a more prolonged protocol with supplementation for 28 days at a rate of 3 g/day elicited about a 20% increase in muscle [TCr], comparable to findings with the more rapid supplementation protocol. At the present time, for those using the more prolonged supplementation protocol, 3 g appears to be the minimum amount. Thompson et al. (1996) reported no beneficial effects on either muscle TCr or PCr levels when supplementing 2 g creatine monohydrate per day for 6 weeks.

Gonzalez de Suso and Prat (1994) found that the subjects whose initial PCr was lower experienced a greater increase in PCr levels after supplementation. Harris et al. (1992) also reported that the effect of creatine supplementation was greatest in subjects with a low initial TCr content and that the effect was to raise the content in these subjects closer to the upper limit of the normal range; in some cases the increase was as much as 50%. In his review, Ekblom (1996) concluded that those subjects who begin with low creatine levels benefit more from the supplementation than those who have high levels when they begin supplementation.

As noted later, even in studies showing significant group increases in muscle [TCr], investigators have observed substantial individual differences. For some reason, there are individuals who do not appear to respond to creatine supplementation to the same degree that others do although consuming a creatine and carbohydrate (glucose) supplement appears to alleviate this problem.

Several principal investigators have indicated that there appears to be a maximal, or optimum, total intracellular creatine concentration of about 150-160 mmol/kg dm (Clark 1997; Greenhaff 1995; Harris et al. 1992), and this maximum occurs in about 20% of subjects (Greenhaff 1996). Summarizing research data, Clark (1997) points to evidence strongly suggesting that there are definite limits to the benefits possible from creatine supplementation, and that once muscle creatine levels have plateaued there will be no further increase. Greenhaff (1997a) also notes that muscle uptake of creatine may be saturated after a standard creatine-loading protocol. Both animal and human studies suggest that extracellular creatine induces the expression of a protein that functionally inactivates creatine transporters—a response that may limit maximal levels (Loike et al. 1988).

There appears to be a maximal, or optimum, total intracellular creatine concentration of about 150-160 mmol/kg dm.

Creatine Supplementation With Carbohydrate   Studies by Green and her colleagues (1996a, 1996b), however, have shown that combining creatine with a simple carbohydrate, such as glucose, will increase creatine transport into the muscle even in subjects with high levels of muscle creatine. In these studies, the solution consisted of 5 g of creatine and about 90 g of simple carbohydrate, consumed four times per day. Both creatine and creatine-carbohydrate supplements increased [TCr] and [PCr], but the creatine-carbohydrate supplement increased [TCr] by 60% and [PCr] by 100% compared to the value with the creatine supplement alone. Also, creatine plus carbohydrate increased the PCr/ATP ratio by 24% compared to 9% for creatine alone. The following data highlight the changes (Green 1996a).

	Creatine		Creatine + carbohydrate		
	Pre	Post	Pre	Post	
PCr	85.1	92.4	84.4	99.4	(100%)
FCr	36.4	49.8	39.0	57.1	(34%)
TCr	121.5	142.2	123.4	156.4	(60%)

Note: Units in mmol/kg dm; % = percentage creatine + carbohydrate increase greater than with creatine alone.

Green and colleagues (1996a) reported that in the creatine-only group, the increase in muscle TCr appeared to be dependent on the initial TCr concentration, as was noted earlier in this chapter. However, this did not appear to be the case in the group receiving both creatine and carbohydrate. One subject who had a particularly high presupplementation TCr concentration (152 mmol/kg dm) experienced a 43 mmol/kg dm increase as a result of the creatine-carbohydrate ingestion, exceeding the postulated maximum amount cited previously.

Combining creatine (5 g) with a simple carbohydrate (90 g), such as glucose, may increase creatine transport into the muscle even in subjects who appear to be less responsive to creatine supplementation.

The investigators suggested that these beneficial effects of a creatine-carbohydrate mixture may be attributed to an insulin-mediated effect. The serum insulin concentration remained constant in the creatine-only group; however, in the creatine-carbohydrate group, the serum insulin concentration increased 17-fold within 20 min of the CHO ingestion. The urinary excretion of creatine was reduced in the creatine-carbohydrate group by nearly 50%, from nearly 10 g to 5 g, suggesting increased creatine retention possibly mediated by insulin.

Creatine Supplementation With Exercise Exercise during the creatine-supplementation period may provide an additive effect relative to muscle creatine uptake. In a creatine-supplement study using a one-leg exercise protocol (Harris et al. 1992), 1 hr of hard exercise per day augmented the increase in the TCr content of the exercised leg, but had no additional effect in the collateral leg. On average, the TCr content went from 118.1 mmol/kg dm at baseline to 148.5 in the control leg and 162.2 in the exercised leg; in one subject, creatine and exercise elevated the creatine content to 182.8 mmol/kg dm, of which 112.0 mmol/kg dm was in the form of PCr.

However, exercise may provide no additional benefit for muscle creatine loading when a creatine-carbohydrate supplement is used. Green and her colleagues (1996b) reported that although carbohydrate ingestion augmented creatine retention during creatine feeding, creatine retention was not further increased when exercise (1 hr cycling at 70% $\dot{V}O_{2max}$) was performed prior to ingestion, at least as compared to the creatine-carbohydrate supplementation protocol.

After the creatine-loading phase, maintenance of elevated muscle creatine levels may be maintained with lower dosages. In their experiment, Hultman et al. (1996) reported that the elevated [TCr] following creatine loading was maintained when supplementation was continued at a rate of only 2 g/day during a 30-day trial. Clark (1996) also indicates that creatine efflux from the muscle cell is considered to be negligible and therefore the concentration of creatine is not at risk of becoming depleted by exercise during this maintenance phase.

Exercise during the creatine-supplementation period may provide an additive effect relative to muscle creatine uptake. However, exercise may provide no additional benefit for muscle creatine loading when a creatine-carbohydrate supplement is used.

Creatine Supplementation With Caffeine   Caffeine is an effective ergogenic aid in its own right (Spriet, 1995). The adrenergic effects of caffeine may elicit a variety of cellular responses, one being an increased sodium/potassium ATPase pump activity in the muscle cell membrane, an effect theorized to enhance muscle creatine uptake. Consequently, consuming caffeine with creatine has been studied to evaluate the effect on intramuscular creatine levels. Vandenberghe et al. (1996a) supplemented young males with either creatine (0.5 g/kg/day) or creatine and caffeine (5 mg/kg/day) for 6 days, evaluating changes in muscle creatine levels by ^{31}P-NMRS. They reported similar increases in muscle PCr approximating 4-6%. In a subsequent study (Vandenberghe et al., 1997b), creatine (25 g/day for 5 days) and creatine plus caffeine (2 × 2.5 mg/kg/day) supplementation again similarly increased muscle PCr by 8-15%, but the rate of muscle PCr resynthesis during intermittent exercise was impaired by the creatine/caffeine combination. Although creatine supplementation alone improved isokinetic dynamometer exercise performance in both of these studies (Vandenberghe et al. 1996a, 1997b), this ergogenic effect was eliminated with the creatine/caffeine supplement protocol. Other research indicates no additional benefit of combining creatine and caffeine supplementation before exercise (Vanakoski et al. 1998).

Muscle Creatine Content Summary   As noted previously, one of the theoretical ergogenic aspects of creatine supplementation is an increase in [TCr] and an enhanced PCr resynthesis during recovery from prior exercise. In their classic study, Greenhaff and his associates (1994a) reported an average 25% increase in TCr at rest, and a mean 19 mmol (35%) increase in PCr resynthesis after electrically evoked isometric muscle contraction; these results provided the first data to indicate that an increase in muscle FCr concentration, resulting from dietary creatine supplementation, can accelerate the rate of muscle PCr resynthesis during recovery from exercise. Findings of increased PCr resynthesis following creatine supplementation, particularly in persons with initially lower resting [PCr], such as aged individuals, were recently confirmed by Smith et al. (1998b).

As an increased muscle concentration of TCr and PCr is the major factor underlying the theoretical ergogenic effect of creatine supplementation, it is important to briefly summarize the findings presented in table 3.2. Most of the studies summarized used the typical creatine-loading protocol (20 g/day for 5-7 days) and employed either muscle biopsies or NMR techniques to analyze muscle creatine content. Twelve studies showed that creatine supplementation increases muscle TCr; nine studies reported increases in PCr; and four studies showed an elevated TCr/β-ATP ratio. In general, individuals with lower muscle creatine levels prior to supplementation experienced greater increases, the average absolute increase in TCr was about 22 mmol/kg dm with a range of 20-27 mmol/kg dm; the average percentage increase was 18.5, with a range of 15-22. The average absolute increase in PCr was about 14.3 mmol/kg dm, with a range of 3.4-26; the average percentage increase was 20.7, with a range of 4-52. The average percentage increase in the TCr/β-ATP ratio was 12, with a range of 6-23. Studies using an indirect measurement (urine creatine content) of creatine retention showed muscle uptake approximating 30-35 g—that is, approximating 38 mmol/kg dm. Several studies provided evidence of enhanced PCr resynthesis following intense exercise. After the loading phase, two studies indicated that elevated creatine levels could be maintained with daily doses approximating 2-5 g.

Several studies showed no significant effect of creatine supplementation on muscle creatine levels. In one investigation, creatine supplementation increased PCr by 6.4 mmol/kg dm, compared to a 2.5 mmol/kg dm increase in the placebo group, but the difference was not statistically significant. In a crossover study, the washout period was only 14 days, which may have confounded the results in that the group supplemented with creatine first would possibly still have had elevated creatine levels when tested during the placebo phase. In yet another study, although the supplementation period was 6 weeks, the daily creatine dose was only 2 g.

Overall, these data provide substantial evidence that creatine supplementation will increase muscle levels of both TCr and PCr.

Studies using the typical creatine-loading protocol have shown an average absolute increase in TCr approximating 22 mmol/kg dm with a range of 20-27 mmol/kg dm; the average percentage increase was 18.5, with a range of 15-22. The average absolute increase in PCr was about 14.3 mmol/kg dm, with a range of 3.4-26; the average percentage increase was 20.7, with a range of 4-52. These data provide substantial evidence that creatine supplementation will increase muscle levels of both TCr and PCr.

Creatine Excretion

As noted in chapter 2, creatine normally is catabolized to creatinine, and this metabolic by-product is excreted by the kidneys. However, the fate of creatine when ingested in large quantities is somewhat different.

Creatine is a low molecular weight compound, and its removal by the kidneys is achieved by diffusion, which is a nonenergy-dependent process. Although most of the orally ingested creatine is absorbed into the body, not all is retained. In their subjects, Harris et al. (1992) reported that renal excretion was 40%, 61%, and 68% of the creatine dose over the first 3 days, indicative of increased excretion rates as body creatine stores increased. Similar findings were reported by Maganaris and Maughan (1998), with an average elimination rate of about 25.5% after the first day of supplementation and an average 48.5% elimination after the fifth day. Poortmans et al. (1997) also reported that creatine supplementation increased urinary creatine content (88.6-fold) as well as creatine clearance (26.1-fold), representing approximately 60% of the oral creatine load. Moreover, no significant differences were seen in urinary creatinine levels or creatinine clearance.

Although almost all orally ingested creatine is absorbed into the body, not all is retained. Most of the absorbed creatine, particularly after the first 2-3 days of loading, is excreted in the urine. About 50-70% is excreted after the second day of loading.

Cessation of Supplementation: Return to Normal Levels

The catabolism of creatine to creatinine—the only means to rid the body of creatine—is a slow process. On the basis of measurements of muscle creatinine excretion, which is known to be increased after creatine ingestion, Greenhaff (1997a) estimated that elevated muscle creatine stores will decline very slowly over 4 weeks following creatine ingestion. Three investigations indicated that muscle creatine levels return to normal in about 28 days, although one study included an individual who still had elevated levels 35 days later. In their longitudinal study of subjects who ingested creatine in different quantities over varying time periods, Hultman et al. (1996) reported that muscle creatine levels returned to normal 30 days after cessation of supplementation.

Effect on Biosynthesis

Under normal dietary conditions, the liver, pancreas, and kidney synthesize about 1 g of creatine per day. In his extensive review of creatine, Walker (1979) cited evidence of the distribution of creatine and creatinine suggesting that exogenous creatine suppressed the biosynthesis of creatine. Greenhaff (1995) recently reiterated this point, but also noted that the depressed biosynthesis is reversible when supplementation ceases. Most likely, creatine supplementation suppresses enzymic activity of amidinotransferase, rather than the methyltransferase reaction, because the former normally controls creatine biosynthesis. However, studies on effects of cessation of creatine supplementation show that it generally takes about 4 to 5 weeks before creatine stores approach initial baseline values (i.e., lose the 20 to 35 g gained from supplementation). Because daily creatine turnover is about 2 g/day, one would expect a greater loss in muscle stores within that period of time if creatine synthesis was totally suppressed by creatine supplementation.

Creatine supplementation appears to depress normal biosynthesis, but this is reversible when supplementation ceases. After cessation of supplementation, elevated muscle creatine stores will decline very slowly to normal over four weeks following creatine ingestion.

Responders and Nonresponders

For some reason, not all individuals who follow standardized creatine-loading protocols increase muscle concentrations of TCr and PCr. As noted earlier, standardized creatine-loading procedures generally increase muscle TCr content by about 25 mmol/kg dry muscle mass—about a 20% increase. Greenhaff (1996) defines nonresponders as those who show less than a 10 mmol/kg dm (8%) increase in muscle TCr following 5 days of 20 g/day. He and his colleagues (Greenhaff et al. 1996) indicated that about 20-30% of individuals do not respond to creatine loading. In one of Greenhaff's studies (1994b), a standard creatine-loading protocol (20 g/day for 5 days) substantially increased muscle [TCr] (mean 29 ± 3 mmol/kg dm) by 25% in five of eight subjects. However, in the remaining three subjects, creatine supplementation had little effect on muscle [TCr], producing increases of 8-9 mmol—about a 5-7% increase. Snow et al. (1998) reported a small, but significant, increase in muscle TCr content following creatine supplementation, but analysis of individual data plots revealed that three subjects were responders (15-20% increase) and five were not (2-10% increase). These investigators had no explanation for the finding that the subjects did not increase muscle TCr as seen in other studies. To optimize chances of muscle creatine retention, creatine and carbohydrate should be supplemented together.

There appear to be substantial individual differences in responses to creatine supplementation, with some individuals being nonresponders (i.e., their muscle creatine concentrations increase only slightly). Consuming creatine with glucose appears to be more effective.

Muscle Creatine Levels and Ergogenic Effects

On the basis of his recent work, Greenhaff (1996, 1997a) believes that it may be necessary to increase muscle TCr concentration by close to or more than 20 mmol/kg dm in order to obtain substantial improvements in exercise performance as a result of creatine supplementation. This may be the case because subjects who increase muscle [TCr] by 20 mmol/kg dm may increase the rate of PCr resynthesis during recovery from exercise (Greenhaff et al. 1994a). Casey et al. (1996) suggest that any performance benefits may be related to increased creatine within the type II muscle fibers.

> Some investigators suggest that in order to obtain an ergogenic effect, one must increase muscle TCr concentration by close to or more than 20 mmol/kg dm, primarily within the type II muscle fibers.

As Greenhaff states (1996), it is clear that subjects vary considerably in the extent of muscle creatine accumulation during supplementation. As noted also by Greenhaff, recent work has revealed that the magnitude of improvement in exercise performance following creatine supplementation is closely associated with the extent of muscle creatine accumulation during supplementation. These findings may provide some insight as to why some individuals do not receive any ergogenic benefits from creatine supplementation.

Chapter Summary

Athletes involved in sports which depend on phosphocreatine (PCr) as a significant contributor to energy production may benefit from increased muscle PCr concentrations. PCr is derived primarily from creatine. Theoretically, dietary creatine supplementation may help prevent fatigue in such athletes by such mechanisms as an increased PCr availability, an increased PCr resynthesis, reduced muscle acidity, enhanced training, and increased body mass. Creatine monohydrate is the most commonly available creatine supplement. Although some individuals are nonresponders, various creatine-loading protocols, particularly those including supplemental carbohydrate, have been shown to increase total muscle creatine (TCr), including free creatine (FCr) and PCr by approximately 20%, a level deemed sufficient to elicit an ergogenic effect.

4

<u>CHAPTER</u>

Research Considerations With Nutritional Sports Ergogenics

All the nutrients in foods we consume are involved in various metabolic processes in the body—many important in energy production for various types of exercise or sport performance. On the basis primarily of the theoretical application of specific nutrients or other dietary constituents to performance enhancement, and given the substantial number of individuals involved in exercise or sport activities, numerous entrepreneurs have developed specific supplements for this segment of the population. The dietary supplement industry has evolved into a worldwide, multibillion dollar business, and increasing numbers of products are being marketed to improve exercise or sport performance. But how do we determine what effect a dietary supplement may have on our exercise or sport performance, or for that matter, on our health?

The answer, of course, is research. Numerous nutrition and exercise and sport science investigators have focused their research efforts on the relationship of various dietary strategies, nutrients, or dietary supplements to exercise and sport performance. They are not only attempting to determine the effect of these nutritional interventions on actual exercise or sport performance, but are also investigating the effects at the cellular and molecular level to ascertain possible mechanisms of action to improve performance. Additionally, some investigators evaluate possible adverse or beneficial health effects of such nutritional interventions. This chapter focuses on the nature and limitations of research strategies used to determine the ergogenic effects, and possible health effects, of dietary supplements marketed to physically active individuals. Experimental research is used to determine the ergogenic effect of a dietary supplement; it may also be used to evaluate health effects, as can epidemiological research.

Research is the key factor in determining the effect a dietary supplement may have on our exercise or sport performance, or for that matter, on our health.

Experimental Research

Experimental research is essential to establishing a cause-and-effect relationship. In such studies, often called intervention studies, an independent variable or variables (cause) are manipulated so that changes in a dependent variable or variables (effect) can be studied. In a study involving the effects of creatine supplementation on isotonic bench press endurance, the independent variable, or cause, would be the creatine supplement, while the dependent variable, or effect, would be the isotonic bench press endurance. Investigators need to define specifically the independent and dependent variable(s). For example, in the bench press study the independent variable (creatine supplementation) could be defined as 20 g/day for 5 days, while the dependent variable (isotonic bench press endurance) could be defined as the number of repetitions at 80% of 1-repetition maximum until exhaustion, as indicated by the inability to complete a full repetition. If the results of this study showed no significant improvement in isotonic bench press endurance, does that mean we can disregard creatine as a useful nutritional ergogenic? Not necessarily, as we shall see later.

Experimental research is essential to establishing a cause-and-effect relationship. In such studies, often called intervention studies, an independent variable or variables (cause) are manipulated so that changes in a dependent variable or variables (effect) can be studied.

Most of the research designed to explore the effect of creatine supplementation on exercise or sport performance is experimental in nature. In chapters 5 through 8, as we discuss the effects of creatine supplementation on various types of exercise or sport performance and body mass and composition, we will often refer to studies that have problems with their experimental methodology but will also note studies that are well controlled. In a recent conference on nutritional ergogenic aids, Sherman and Lamb (1995) listed the principal standards for experimental approaches to research with nutritional ergogenics such as dietary supplements. The following are some of the major questions one should ask to evaluate the experimental methodology of a study involving the effect of dietary supplements on exercise or sport performance in order to determine whether the investigation has been well designed. We shall use research with creatine supplementation and its effect on muscular power, achieved through resistance training, as an example.

Most of the research designed to explore the effect of creatine supplementation on exercise or sport performance is experimental in nature.

---

1. Is there a legitimate reason for creatine supplementation? Theoretically, creatine may add to the stores of total creatine (TCr) and phosphocreatine (PCr) in the muscle, an important energy source for high muscular power. The creatine dosage should be one that has been reported to increase TCr stores.
2. Were appropriate subjects used? As one of the purported effects of increased PCr is increased muscular power, trained strength athletes would be ideal subjects.
3. Are the performance tests valid? Validated tests should be used to collect data on the dependent variable, in this case valid muscular power tests, such as various isokinetic protocols. Subjects should be familiarized with the performance tests before the experimentation period.
4. Have underlying mechanisms been evaluated? As the major underlying premise for increased muscle power with creatine supplementation is an increased muscle PCr content, was the muscle PCr measured?
5. Was a placebo control used? A placebo, similar in appearance and taste to creatine, should be used.
6. Were the subjects randomly assigned to treatments? Subjects should be randomly assigned to the treatment (creatine) or the control (placebo) group.
7. Was the study double-blind? Neither the investigators nor the subjects should know which groups received the treatment or placebo until the conclusion of the study. One possible side effect of creatine supplementation is a rapid weight gain, which may interfere with a double-blind protocol.
8. Was a repeated-measures, crossover design used? In a repeated-measures design, in which all subjects take both the creatine and placebo in different trials after a washout period, the order of administration of the creatine and placebo is counterbalanced; this is known as a crossover design. This design helps minimize variation between subjects. As muscle creatine levels following supplementation may decrease slowly, at least a 4-week washout period should be used.
9. Were extraneous factors controlled? Investigators should try to control other factors that may influence power, such as physical training, diet (including caffeine), and activity prior to testing.
10. Were the data analyzed properly? Appropriate statistical techniques should be used to reduce the risk of statistical error. Using a reasonable number of subjects also helps to increase statistical power and minimize statistical error.

Creatine Supplementation Study Conditions

Well-controlled studies investigating the effects of creatine supplementation on various types of exercise or sport performance, body mass and composition, and health status usually adhere to most of the following conditions:

a. Use of exercise- or sport-trained subjects
b. Use of valid and reliable performance tests
c. Use of a placebo control
d. Random assignment of subjects to treatments
e. Use of a double-blind protocol
f. Control of extraneous factors
g. Use of proper statistical analyses

Although not many studies addressing the ergogenic effect of dietary supplements adhere to all of these experimental standards, most experienced contemporary investigators generally use similar sophisticated research designs to generate meaningful data. However, some researchers do not apply such strict protocols and thus may produce erroneous conclusions.

Experimental research may also be used to evaluate the short-term effect of dietary supplements on health status, using research designs comparable to those in studies investigating the effects on exercise or sport performance. For example, because the kidney is the major body organ involved in the excretion of creatinine, the metabolic by-product of creatine, experimental protocols may be used to evaluate the effects of short-term creatine supplementation on kidney function.

Epidemiological Research

Evaluation of the long-term effects of dietary supplements on health status is most commonly achieved with epidemiological research. Epidemiological research helps scientists identify important relationships between nutritional practices and health. One general form uses retrospective techniques. In a group case-study approach, individuals who have a particular disease, such as kidney disease, are identified and compared with a group of their peers, called a cohort, who do not have the disease. Researchers then trace the history of both groups through interviewing techniques in attempts to identify dietary practices that may have increased the risk for developing the disease. If it were to be found that the group with kidney disease used creatine supplements significantly more than the group without the disease, this might suggest a relationship between creatine supplementation and renal malfunction. However, one should note that such research does not prove a cause-and-effect relationship. Although such a retrospective study might note a deleterious association between creatine supplementation and renal function, it does not actually prove that creatine supplementation contributes to kidney problems. Unfortunately, widespread creatine supplementation is a rather recent phenomenon, and it generally takes substantial time for chronic health problems such as kidney disease to develop, so currently we have limited epidemiological data regarding any adverse health effects of chronic creatine supplementation on large numbers of individuals—although some clinical and individual case-study data are available.

Evaluation of the long-term effects of dietary supplements on health status is most commonly achieved with epidemiological research. Epidemiological research helps scientists identify important relationships between nutritional practices and chronic health problems.

Another source of epidemiological data is the Special Nutritionals Adverse Event Monitoring System, a project of the U.S. Food and Drug Administration (FDA), Center for Food Safety and Applied Nutrition, Office of Special Nutritionals. The sources of information for this project are reports of adverse events (illness or injury) associated with use of a special nutritional product, such as dietary supplements; the information comes from FDA field offices, from other federal, state, and local public health agencies, and from letters and phone calls from health professionals and consumers. Although some adverse events have been reported in association with creatine supplementation, the FDA cautions that there is no certainty that a reported adverse event can be attributed to a particular product or ingredient, for the available information may not be complete enough to allow that determination. Individually these reports may be considered to be anecdotal evidence and may be grounds for a concerted research effort to explore the relationship, particularly if there are multiple reports of similar circumstances. The reader may access this website at **http://vm.cfsan.fda.gov/~dms/aems.html** to uncover reports of adverse events associated with use of dietary supplements.

Widespread creatine supplementation is a rather recent phenomenon, and it generally takes substantial time for chronic health problems to develop, so currently we have limited epidemiological data regarding any adverse health effects of chronic creatine supplementation on large numbers of individuals.

One form of epidemiological research involves an experimental approach whereby, over a long time frame, a significantly large population is exposed to a dietary supplement while another group receives a placebo, and the health effects are determined periodically until the completion of the intervention period. There appear to be no available data based on this approach. However, one of the purported adverse side effects of creatine supplementation among athletes is an increased incidence of muscle cramps or muscle strains, and this relationship is currently being studied by the National Collegiate Athletic Association using this research approach. A related approach is an open-label study, in which one group of subjects knowingly takes a supplement while a control group does not. Some safety data using this research protocol are presented in chapter 9.

Research-Based Recommendations

Research evaluating the effect of dietary supplements on exercise or sport performance in human subjects is difficult. It is not easy to control all the factors that may influence exercise or sport performance on any given day in freely living human beings so that we can isolate one independent variable, such as creatine supplementation, and determine its ergogenic effect. Numerous physiological, psychological, and biomechanical factors influence physical performance on any given day. Why cannot athletes match their personal records day after day, such as the recent 2:06:05 world-record marathon performance by Ronaldo da Costa from Brazil? The answer is that their physiology and psychology vary from day to day, and even within the day. So it is with subjects, either trained or untrained, who participate in dietary supplement studies.

Nevertheless, it is these individual studies that provide us with the basis for making recommendations regarding the efficacy of purported nutritional ergogenic aids, so it is important that we furnish the rationale underlying the inclusion of studies incorporated in this monograph.

The published details regarding methods and results of individual studies may be presented in a variety of formats, but the two most prevalent are abstracts of studies presented at scientific meetings and peer-reviewed (reviewed by several other experts) articles in scientific journals. When an ample number of these individual studies have been published, a review article may be published and a conclusion possibly rendered regarding the efficacy of the dietary supplement as an ergogenic aid. When a substantial number of individual studies have been published, a statistical analysis of the studies known as a meta-analysis may be performed.

Research evaluating the effect of dietary supplements on exercise or sport performance in human subjects is difficult. Nevertheless, individual studies provide us with the basis for making recommendations regarding the efficacy of purported nutritional ergogenic aids.

This book incorporates information from published abstracts, peer-reviewed articles, and reviews. Although a well-written abstract may provide enough information to document the effect of creatine supplementation, it does not provide the same level of detail as a peer-reviewed article. We have included abstracts in our book if they have provided us with essential information relative to the subjects, the supplementation protocol, the major dependent variables, the statistics, and the conclusions. We also considered the reputation of the research laboratory conducting the investigation. When certain details were missing, authors were contacted by telephone or email so that the necessary information could be obtained. Often, these investigators would provide a copy of the unpublished manuscript so that we could analyze the details.

Although well-designed studies in peer-reviewed scientific journals serve as the basis for an informed decision as to whether a dietary supplement enhances exercise or sport performance, it is important to realize that the results of one study do not prove anything. Although most investigators attempt to control extraneous factors that may interfere with interpretation of the results of their study, there may be some unknown factor that leads to an erroneous conclusion.

To truly evaluate the effect of dietary supplements on exercise or sport performance, individual studies need to be repeated by other scientists and, if possible, a consensus needs to be developed. Reviews provide a stronger foundation than the results of an individual study. In reviews, an investigator analyzes most or all of the research on a particular topic and usually offers a summary and conclusion. However, the conclusion may be influenced by the studies reviewed or by the reviewer's orientation.

Meta-analysis, a review process that involves a statistical analysis of previously published studies, may actually provide a quantification and the strongest evidence available relative to the effect of dietary supplements on exercise or sport performance. Unfortunately, at the time of this writing, no meta-analysis of the effects of creatine supplementation on exercise or sport performance has been performed.

The conclusions and recommendations presented in this book are based on an analysis of approximately 70 published research abstracts, 80 published studies, and 35 reviews in which the effects of creatine supplementation on various aspects of exercise or sport performance and health have been analyzed. Many studies evaluated the effect of creatine supplementation on multiple dependent variables, so the same study may be cited several times.

Chapter Summary

Research is the key factor to evaluate the ergogenic efficacy or health effects of creatine supplementation and, subsequently, to present recommendations. Well-designed experimental research is essential to establishing a cause-and-effect relationship relative to performance or health, while epidemiological research helps identify important relationships between creatine supplementation and chronic health problems. Numerous experimental studies have evaluated the effect of creatine supplementation on exercise performance, while fewer experimental and epidemiological studies have evaluated its health effects. The conclusions and recommendations presented in this monograph are based on an analysis of currently available research, including approximately 70 published abstracts, 80 peer-reviewed articles, and 35 reviews focusing on the various exercise performance and health effects of creatine supplementation.

5

CHAPTER

Ergogenic Effects of Creatine Supplementation on Anaerobic Power

As discussed in chapter 3, the source of adenosine triphosphate (ATP) for performance of single or repetitive high-intensity, short-duration tasks (anaerobic power) is stored ATP and rapid rephosphorylation of adenosine diphosphate (ADP) by phosphocreatine (PCr). Theoretically, the phosphagen, or ATP-PCr, energy system is capable of providing ATP for only a few muscle contractions before being depleted. Since PCr is the substrate for this system, it is logical to hypothesize that creatine supplementation is a possible ergogenic strategy to rapidly increase PCr or replenish PCr to phosphorylate ADP during and following such exercise. Indeed, the majority of investigations have focused on high-intensity repetitive and/or single-bout exercise in which the performance task is less than or equal to 30 sec in duration.

Theoretically, the phosphagen, or ATP-PCr, energy system is capable of providing ATP for only a few muscle contractions before being depleted. Since PCr is the substrate for this system, it is logical to hypothesize that creatine supplementation is a possible ergogenic strategy to rapidly replenish PCr and enhance performance in exercise tasks less than or equal to 30 sec in duration.

This chapter reviews studies involving the effects of creatine monohydrate supplementation on laboratory-based muscular strength and endurance, and various cycling task protocols, as well as field-based tasks such as running, jumping, and swimming. Tables 5.1 to 5.8 present the key points of these studies, with more details as available presented in the text. Unless otherwise indicated, all investigations employed a double-blind placebo control design. The length of the washout period, the importance of which has been discussed previously, is provided in studies using a crossover design. When possible, *within-group* percentage changes (supplemented group or condition prescore vs. postscore) in performance (either reported by the investigators or calculated from the available data as $[(post-pre)\div pre\cdot 100])$ are provided. Percentage change in a repetitive exercise protocol was calculated using the pre- and postsupplementation performances for the last bout.

Although muscle (creatine) was not measured in most studies, the method (e.g., biopsy, ^{31}P-magnetic resonance spectroscopy (^{31}P-MRS), urinary creatine/creatinine excretion) is indicated for those studies which did measure creatine uptake. It is important to note that some studies which measured more than one dependent variable (e.g., multiple measures of muscular strength and/or endurance) report both ergogenic and nonergogenic findings, whereas other studies which investigated different doses or forms of creatine ingestion also report both ergogenic and nonergogenic findings. Finally, studies which included biochemical markers of energy metabolism in addition to performance variables (e.g., measurement of blood [lactate], [NH$_3$], [hypoxanthine]) also will be discussed.

Of 80 studies addressing the effect of creatine supplementation on performance of activities that rely primarily on the ATP-PCr energy system, 50 revealed beneficial ergogenic effects. Performance modes that appear to be more favorably affected include repetitive cycle ergometry (18 [75%] of 24 studies), isokinetic torque production (7 [50%] of 14 studies), and isotonic force production (17 [74%] of 23 studies). These significant results were obtained almost exclusively in a laboratory environment. An ergogenic effect of creatine was reported in 9 of the 19 (47%) field studies reviewed here.

Laboratory Studies

Numerous researchers have investigated the effect of creatine supplementation on exercise tasks dependent primarily on the ATP-PCr energy system, particularly isometric, isotonic, and isokinetic exercise tasks and various cycle ergometer protocols.

Numerous laboratory studies have addressed the effect of creatine supplementation on exercise tasks dependent primarily on the ATP-PCr energy system, particularly isometric, isotonic, and isokinetic exercise tasks and various cycle ergometer protocols.

Isometric Strength and Endurance

Investigations of the ergogenic effect of creatine on isometric force production are presented in table 5.1. The studies in this section are discussed relative to the effects of supplementation. Of the nine studies reviewed in this section, five reported significant improvement (mean = 27%; median = 19%), while four studies showed no beneficial effect. No studies showed any ergolytic effect on isometric performance following creatine supplementation.

Studies Reporting Ergogenic Effects   Investigating the effects of creatine supplementation on a clinical population, Andrews et al. (1998) randomly assigned congestive heart failure patients to either a placebo or creatine (20 g/day for 5 days, 100 g total) group. Before and after supplementation, patients' maximal voluntary handgrip strength was measured, as well as the number of contractions performed at 25%, 50%, and 75% of maximal voluntary isometric grip strength (5 sec contraction with a 5 sec rest). Creatine supplementation resulted in a 75% increase in the median number of contractions performed (pre- = 8 vs. post- = 14). The authors concluded that creatine supplementation augments skeletal muscle endurance and attenuates the abnormal skeletal muscle responses typically seen in congestive heart failure patients.

In a single-group repeated-measures study combining creatine supplementation with isometric training, Kurosawa et al. (1997) trained five male and female subjects using a 2-week isometric grip exercise protocol. During six sessions per day, subjects trained the nondominant forearm isometrically to exhaustion at a rate of 1 contraction per second at 30% of maximal voluntary contraction; they also consumed 5 g creatine monohydrate per day (70 g total). Prior to and following training, high-intensity (measured in Newton meters per second (Nm/sec) and low-intensity grip performances (time to exhaustion using the training protocol) were measured in both the dominant and the nondominant arm. Following supplementation, forearm muscle [PCr], measured by ^{31}P-MRS, was significantly increased in both arms. In addition, high-intensity grip strength improved significantly in both the nontrained (2.2 Nm/sec, 20%) and the trained (3.2 Nm/sec, 35%) arms. The authors concluded that 2 weeks of creatine supplementation increased muscle [PCr] and enhanced high-intensity exercise performance.

Lemon et al. (1995) studied the effect of creatine monohydrate supplementation (20 g/day for 5 days, 100 g total) on total integrated force in 20 × 30 sec maximal isometric ankle extensions with a 16 sec recovery between contractions. A crossover design was employed, with seven males as subjects. The washout period was 5 weeks. Creatine supplementation increased the preexercise muscle [PCr]/[ß-ATP] ratio and significantly increased total integrated muscle force by 11%.

In another crossover design, Maganaris and Maughan (1998) studied the effects of placebo and creatine supplementation (10 g/day for 5 days, 50 g total) on isometric knee extensor strength in 10 healthy males involved in resistance training. The 5-day supplementation periods were separated by a washout period of only 3 days. Urinalysis revealed that approximately 18 g (35%) of the ingested creatine

Table 5.1 Effect of Creatine Supplementation on High-Intensity, Short-Duration (≤ 30 sec) Single or Repetitive Isometric (IM) Resistive Exercise Performance Tasks Involving the Adenosine Triphosphate-Phosphocreatine (ATP-PCr) Energy System. Studies Are Arranged Alphabetically.

Investigator	Year	Population	N	Gender	Design	Initial CM dose $g \times d = dose$			Mode	Ergogenic effect?	%Δ	Comments
Andrews et al.	1998	Congestive heart failure patients	20	M	RDBPC	20	5	100	75% of maximal contraction 5 sec contraction w/ 5 sec rest	Y	75	Median number of contractions performed increased from 8 to 14 after supplementation.
Bermon et al.	1998	Elderly	32	M/F	RDBPC	20 3	5 47	100 141	Leg extension/ chest press	N		
Kurosawa et al.	1997	Healthy	5	M/F	SGRM	5	14	70	Grip strength with training	Y	20	Increase in nontrained arm; 35% increase in trained arm.
Lemon et al.	1995	Physically active	7	M	RDBPCX	20	5	100	Ankle extensions (20 × 30 sec max)	Y	11	Increase in total and maximal force production.

Maganaris and Maughan	1998	Healthy	10	M	RDBPCX	10	5	50	Knee extensor MVC	Y	10	Increase in both legs (850 N dominant; 800 N nondominant). Group receiving creatine first had residual effects in placebo trial due to inadequate washout.
Tarnopolsky et al.	1997	Patients with exercise intolerance	7	M/F	RDBPCX	10	14	140	Grip strength/ endurance	Y	19	Increase at 10 and 40 sec, but no effect on maximal voluntary force.
Rawson et al.	1998	Older	16	M	RDBPC	20	5	100	Forearm flexors	N		
Stevenson and Dudley	1998	Resistance trained	19	M	RDBPC	20	7	140	MVC knee flexion 45°	N		
Vandenberghe et al.	1996a	Healthy	9	M	RDBPCX	40	6	240	Maximal knee extension (x 3)	N		

MVC = Maximal voluntary contraction

SGRM = Single group, repeated measures

RDBPC = Randomized, double-blind, placebo control

RDBPCX = Randomized, double-blind, placebo control, crossover

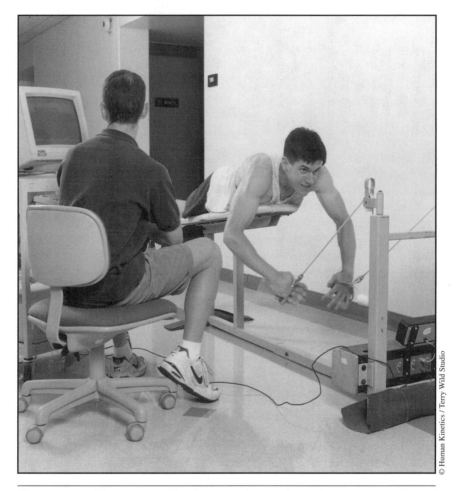

Figure 5.1 Isokinetic testing has been used to evaluate the ergogenic effect of creatine supplementation.

was excreted during the supplementation. Creatine supplementation resulted in a 10% increase in isometric strength of both legs. Examination of the data showed that the group receiving creatine as their first treatment retained the improvements in isometric strength during the placebo treatment. The authors suggested that muscle hypertrophy in response to creatine supplementation during resistance training may explain their results.

Studying creatine supplementation in a clinical population, Tarnopolsky et al. (1997) employed a crossover design to investigate the effects of creatine on grip strength and force production in seven patients with severe exercise intolerance. The patients, who had resting blood [lactate] ≥ 2.7 mmol/L, were supplemented with 10 g/day of creatine monohydrate for 14 days (140 g total). Increases in sustained grip strength were observed at 10 and 40 sec, but there was no change in maximal voluntary isometric grip strength.

Van Leemputte et al. (1999) recently studied the effect of creatine supplementation (5 g/day for 5 days) on contraction and relaxation times in 12 maximal isometric 3-sec elbow flexions interspersed with 10-sec rest intervals. They reported that creatine supplementation decreased the relaxation times by about 20%, which could be the underlying mechanism creating the potential ergogenic effect during interval muscle contractions.

Studies Reporting No Ergogenic Effects   In contrast, four other studies reported no significant effects of creatine supplementation on isometric strength or endurance. Bermon et al. (1998) randomly assigned 32 elderly male and female subjects between 67 and 80 years of age to one of four groups: sedentary-placebo; sedentary-creatine; training-placebo; and training-creatine. Intermittent isometric performance (12 × 12 sec contractions with 3 sec rest) was measured using a force transducer with a 5 millisecond resolution before and after an 8-week supplementation period (20 g/day for 5 days [100 g], followed by 3 g/day for 47 days [141 g, 241 g total]). During this period the training groups completed three sets of eight repetitions at 80 percent of one-repetition maximum (1-RM) in leg press, leg extension, and chest press exercises 3 days/week. Dependent variables included measurement of force over time and the percent force decrement, calculated as the highest force in the first three contractions minus the highest force in the last contraction. Data were normalized to Newtons per kilogram of lean body mass (N/kg LBM). There were no creatine, training, or interaction (supplementation by training) effects on isometric force or percent force decrement for chest press, leg press, or leg extension force exercises. The authors concluded that creatine supplementation alone or in combination with training was ineffective in improving isometric force production or fatigue resistance in healthy, elderly subjects.

Another study involving a geriatric population was conducted by Rawson et al. (1998). Sixteen males (60-78 years of age) were assigned to either a placebo or acute supplementation (20 g/day for 5 days, 100 g total) group. Isometric strength of the forearm flexor muscles was not improved by creatine supplementation. Stevenson and Dudley (1998) assigned 19 resistance-trained male subjects to a placebo or creatine supplementation (20 g/day for 7 days, 140 g total) group in order to investigate the effects of creatine on isometric strength. Supplementation did not significantly increase lower extremity isometric strength at 45° of knee flexion. In a crossover design, Vandenberghe et al. (1996a) measured maximal static (isometric) quadriceps force production at joint angles of 95°, 120°, and 145° in nine healthy males who received both placebo and supplementation (40 g/day for 6 days, 240 g total) with a 3-week washout period. No improvement in isometric force production was observed at any of these joint angles following creatine supplementation.

Summary   The available literature on isometric performance following creatine supplementation is somewhat equivocal. Nevertheless, the majority of studies report an ergogenic effect following creatine supplementation. Although isometric force production is a convenient laboratory-based methodology, perhaps a contributing factor to the paucity of studies is the limited application of isometric force production to actual sport performance.

Of nine studies that have evaluated the effect of creatine supplementation on isometric strength/endurance, five showed significant improvements (mean = 27% for five of the six studies; median = 19%), while four studies showed no beneficial effect. No studies showed any ergolytic effect on isometric performance following creatine supplementation.

Isotonic Strength and Endurance

Studies of the effect of creatine on isotonic strength are presented in table 5.2. Of 23 studies, 17 showed improvements (mean 15% for 11 of the 17 studies; median = 9%) in various measures of isotonic strength and endurance following creatine supplementation. Eight studies showed no beneficial effect after creatine supplementation, and no studies showed an ergolytic effect. Of the eight studies, two (Goldberg and Bechtel, 1997; Stout et al., 1999) reported both ergogenic and no ergogenic effects.

Studies Reporting Ergogenic Effects   Becque et al. (1997) investigated the effect of creatine-supplemented strength training (6-week periodized program beginning with 8-repetition maximum [RM] and ending with 2-RM) on 1-RM performance. Twenty-three experienced male weight lifters were assigned in a double-blind, *non*randomized manner to either a creatine-supplementation (20 g/day for 7 days, 140 g total) or placebo (sucrose) group. Following the initial loading regimen, the creatine-supplementation group also received a maintenance regimen (2 g/day for 35 days, 70 g total). Strength training significantly increased 1-RM strength in both groups, but the creatine-supplemented group experienced greater increases in 1-RM strength than the placebo group.

Earnest et al. (1995) randomly assigned eight weight-trained males to either placebo control or creatine supplementation (20 g/day for 14 days, 280 g total) in a double-blind manner. Significant increases in bench press 1-RM (6%) and bench press repetitions at 70% of 1-RM (35%) were observed in the creatine group.

Kelly and Jenkins (1998) randomly assigned 18 male trained weight lifters to either placebo or creatine supplementation (20 g/day for 5 days, 100 g total). Following this initial loading regimen, supplemented subjects received an additional 5 g/day for 21 days (105 g total). Dependent variables included 3-RM and five sets of 85% 1-RM repetitions to fatigue. Increases in 3-RM were observed in both groups, but the increase was significantly greater in the creatine group. The creatine group also significantly increased the number of repetitions in all five sets compared to no change in the placebo group. The authors concluded that 26 days of creatine supplementation improves strength and near-maximal bench press performance.

Table 5.2 Effect of Creatine Supplementation on High-Intensity, Short-Duration (≤ 30 sec) Single or Repetitive Isotonic (IT) Resistive Exercise Performance Tasks Involving the Adenosine Triphosphate-Phosphocreatine (ATP-PCr) Energy System. Studies Are Arranged According to Ergogenic Effect.

Investigator	Year	Population	N	Gender	Design	Initial CM dose g × d = dose		Mode	Ergogenic effect?	%Δ	Comments
Becque et al.	1997	Weight lifters	23	M	RDBPC	7	20 140	1-RM bicep curl	Y	28	Comparison of CM powder vs. gum. No real control group, so ergogenic effect is uncertain.
Crowder et al.	1998	Lightweight football players	31	M	RDBPC	5	3 15	1-RM power clean, squat, bench press	Y	N/A	
Earnest et al.	1995	Weight trained	8	M	RDBPC	20	14 280	1-RM bench press; reps at 70% 1-RM	Y	6	1-RM increased 6%; # of reps increased 35%.
Kelly and Jenkins	1998	Trained weight lifters	18	M	RDBPC	20 5	5 100 21 105	3-RM bench press; 85% 1-RM × 5 sets to fatigue	Y	7.8	3-RM increased in both PL and CM, but more so in CM. Increased reps in all 5 sets in CM group.
Knehans et al.	1998	Football players	25	M	RDBPC	20 3	5 100 58 174	1-RM bench press, squat, power clean	Y Y	4.9 8	

(continued)

Table 5.2 *(continued)*

Investigator	Year	Population	N	Gender	Design	Initial CM dose g × d = dose			Mode	Ergogenic effect?	%Δ	Comments
Kreider et al.	1998b	NCAA IA football players	25	M	RDBPC	15.75	28	441	1-RM bench press, squat, power clean	Y	40	Increase in total lift volume was greater for CM than PL group.
Larson et al.	1998	Soccer players	14	F	RDBPC	15 5	7 60	105 300	1-RM bench press	Y	N/A	12 wk maintenance dose of 5 g/d followed initial regimen. Strength increased at 3-5 wk, with no further change.
Noonan et al.	1998b	College athletes	39	M	RDBPC	20	5	100	1-RM bench press	Y	5.8	Comparison of two doses 100mg/kg (8.5 g/d) vs. 300 mg/kg (25.5 g/d). Improvement with both doses.
Pearson et al.	1998	Football players	16	M	RDBPC	5	70	350	1-RM bench press, squat	Y Y	3.4 21.5	5.1 kg bench press increase. 31.5 kg squat increase.
Peeters et al.	1999	Strength trained	35	M	RDBPC	20 10	3 42	60 420	1-RM bench, leg press; reps to fatigue	Y	9.6	Comparison of CM and creatine phosphate (CP). Bench press improved at 3 wk

Study	Year	Subjects	N	Sex	Design				Measure	Sig	%	Results
										Y	8.5	but not leg press or reps for CM. Compared to PL, performance was constant or improved at 6 wk for CM.
												Comparison of creatine phosphate (CP) and CM. Bench press improved at 3 wk, but not leg press or reps for CP. Compared to PL, performance was constant or improved at 6 wk for CP.
Stone et al.	1999	Football players	42	M	RDBPC	20	35	700	1-RM bench and squat	Y Y	10 11.6	Increase of 10.9% for combined bench (124.5 to 136.9 kg) and squat (149 to 167 kg).
Stone et al.	1999	Football players	42	M	RDBPC	8	35	280	1-RM bench and squat	Y Y	10.2 8.9	Increase of 9.1% for combined bench (113.6 to 125.2 kg) and squat (149 to 162 kg).

(continued)

Table 5.2 *(continued)*

Investigator	Year	Population	N	Gender	Design	Initial CM dose g × d = dose			Mode	Ergogenic effect?	%Δ	Comments
Stout et al.	1999	Football players	24	M	RDBPC	21	5	105	1-RM bench press	Y	N/A	Increase in bench press 1-RM by 28.8 kg with Phosphagen HP™ compared to placebo gain of 13.1 kg during training.
Volek et al.	1999	Resistance trained	19	M	RDBPC	25 5	7 77	175 385	1-RM bench press and squat	Y	24 32	Bench and squat increased after 12 wk; bench press increased 5% after 7 d.
Volek et al.	1997a	Healthy active	14	M	RDBPC	25	7	175	Bench press; jump squat	Y	28	Increased bench press reps 5 × 10 and jump squat power.
Vukovich and Michaelis	1999	Males	48	M	RDBPC	20 10	5 16	100 160	1-RM leg press	Y	N/A	Comparison of creatine powder (63.1 kg increase) and creatine candy (52.9 kg increase); placebo no significant change.
Warber et al.	1998	U.S. soldiers	25	M	RDBPC	24	5	120	Bench press (5 sets to failure at 70% of 1-RM)	Y	14.4	Increase in total reps performed over the 5 sets.

Reference	Year	Population	Age	Sex	Design				Measurement	Significance
Bermon et al.	1998	Elderly	32	M/F	RDBPC	20 / 3	5 / 47	100 / 141	Chest press, leg press, leg extension	N
Goldberg and Bechtel	1997	Varsity football and track athletes	34	M	RDBPC	3	14	42	1-RM bench press	N
Hamilton-Ward et al.	1997	Athletes	20	F	RDBPC	25	7	175	1-RM elbow flexion	N
Stevenson and Dudley	1998	Resistance trained	19	M	RDBPC	20	7	140	1-RM knee extension; 5 sets of knee extension at 55% of 1-RM	N
Stout et al.	1999	Football players	24	M	RDBPC	21	5	105	1-RM bench, press	N
Syrotuik et al.	1998	Untrained subjects undergoing resistance training	21	M	RDBPC	20 / 2	5 / 32	100 / 64	1-RM bench, leg press; 50% 1-RM bench and inclined leg press to failure.	N
Wood et al.	1998	Weight trained	44	M	RDBPC	20 / 2	5 / 37	100 / 74	1-RM bench press	N

CM = creatine monohydrate
PL = placebo
RDBPC = Randomized, double-blind, placebo control

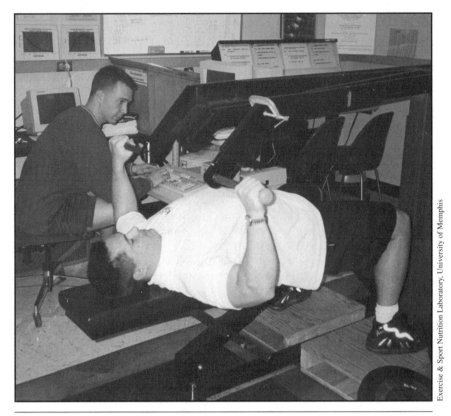

Exercise & Sport Nutrition Laboratory, University of Memphis

Figure 5.2 Lifting weights, an isotonic exercise, is an effective means to evaluate the ergogenic effect of creatine that may have a direct application to sport performance.

Knehans et al. (1998) randomly assigned 25 American football players who were currently undergoing resistance training to either a placebo or creatine group. Supplementation consisted of an initial loading phase of 20 g/day for 5 days (100 g total) followed by a maintenance regimen of 3 g/day for 58 days (174 g total). Bench press and squat 1-RM were measured prior to and after supplementation. Improvements of 4.9% and 8% were reported in bench press and squat 1-RM, respectively, following creatine supplementation. The authors concluded that creatine supplementation may benefit athletes who are also involved in resistance training.

In another study of American football players, Kreider et al. (1998b) matched 25 National Collegiate Athletic Association (NCAA) Division IA players on body mass and randomly assigned them to a group receiving a commercial dietary supplement (Phosphagain™) either without (placebo) or with creatine (15.75 g/day for 28 days, 441 g total). Dependent variables included improvement in 1-RM bench press, squat, power clean, and total lifting volume. Although supplementation did not improve 1-RM for the individual exercises, the improvement in total lifting volume was 40% greater after creatine supplementation compared to placebo.

In one of the few studies supporting the ergogenicity of creatine in females, Larson et al. (1998) assigned 14 soccer players to either placebo or acute supplementation (15 g/day for 7 days, 105 g total). After the initial loading regimen, creatine subjects received an additional 5 g/day for 60 days (300 g total). The authors reported increased bench press strength at 3-5 weeks after baseline, with no further improvements at 13 weeks. It would appear that in these subjects, improvement in isotonic strength following creatine ingestion was linked to the acute loading regimen and not associated with chronic supplementation.

After an initial loading regimen (20 g/day for 5 days, 100 g total), Noonan et al. (1998b) compared the effects of two maintenance supplementation doses (8 weeks of either 100 mg/kg [~8.5 g/day, 470 g total] or 300 mg/kg [~25.5 g/day, 1,400 g total]) on isotonic strength in 39 male college athletes. These maintenance doses were based on fat-free mass. Bench press 1-RM improved by 5.8% in both supplementation groups, with no difference between groups.

Pearson et al. (1998) investigated the effects of a low-dose (5 g/day) chronic supplementation regimen (70 days, 350 g total) vs. placebo on bench press, squat, and power clean 1-RM in 16 American football players who were also participating in resistance training. After supplementation, increases were observed in bench press (2.3 kg, 3.4%), squat (9.8 kg, 31.5%), and power clean 1-RM performance. Upon examination of the data, it appears that the creatine group was somewhat stronger at baseline. The difference in strength between the groups at baseline is presumably why ANCOVA was used to analyze the data. It is interesting to note that resistance training failed to improve isotonic strength in the placebo group. According to the authors' speculation, the reason for this observation may have been that the resistance training regimen offered either too little overload (insufficient stimulus for improvement) or too much overload (overtraining). In the case of the latter possibility, the authors speculated that creatine supplementation might serve as a protection against overtraining.

Stone et al. (1999) randomly assigned 42 American collegiate freshman football players to one of four groups. One group received a high-dose creatine supplement (0.22 g/kg body mass per day [~20 g/day] for 35 days, ~700 g total), while a separate group received a supplement containing a lower dose of creatine (0.09 g/kg body mass per day [~8 g/day] for 35 days, ~280 g total) which also contained pyruvate. The other two groups received either an anhydrous water-soluble powder or silica as placebos. Prior to and after the 5-week supplementation regimen, bench press and squat 1-RM was measured on all subjects. The high- and low-dose creatine groups increased total lifting volume by 10.9% and 9.1%, respectively, compared to presupplementation values. Specifically, the high-dose group increased bench press and squat 1-RM by 10% (124.5 to 136.9 kg) and 11.6% (149.7 to 167 kg), respectively. The low-dose group increased bench press and squat 1-RM by 10.2% (114 to 125 kg) and 8.9% (149 to 162 kg). Total lifting volume did not change significantly in either of the placebo groups.

Volek et al. (1997b) assigned 14 healthy, active males in a double-blind manner to either a placebo or creatine-supplementation (25 g/day for 7 days, 175 g total) group. Dependent variables were bench press performance (five sets to failure using a 10-RM resistance) and jump squat performance (five sets of 10 repetitions using 30% of squat 1-RM). Creatine supplementation significantly increased power output in the number of 10-RM bench press repetitions (28%) and all five jump squat sets.

In a recent study of isotonic strength and endurance by Volek et al. (1999), 19 healthy resistance-trained males were randomly assigned to either a placebo or creatine supplementation (25 g/day for 7 days, 175 g total), followed by 5 g/day for the next 11 weeks (385 g, ~560 g total). Total muscle [creatine], measured by biopsy, was increased by 22% (122.9 to 149.9 mmol/kg dm) after one week of supplementation. At 12 weeks, total muscle [creatine] remained significantly increased in the creatine group compared to both baseline (135. 9 mmol/kg dm, 11%) and to the placebo group (19%). Subjects participated in a periodized heavy-resistance training throughout the study. Following one week of supplementation, 1-RM squat performance was not significantly changed in either group. After 12 weeks, however, a 32% increase in 1-RM squat performance was observed in the creatine group (142.1 kg) compared to baseline (107.8 kg). The placebo group also increased 1-RM squat performance (109.5 to 135.3 kg, 24%) at 12 weeks. Creatine supplementation significantly increased bench press 1-RM from 93.0 kg (baseline) to 98.0 kg (5%, week 1) to 115.6 kg (24%, week 12). In the placebo group, the increase in 1-RM bench press was significant at week 12 (109.9 kg, 16%) compared to baseline (94.9 kg). At 12 weeks, bench press and squat 1-RM performances were significantly greater in the creatine group compared to the placebo group. There was no significant change in upper body isotonic endurance, measured as the number of bench press repetitions at 80% of 1-RM, in either group at any time in the study. The authors concluded that the increase in upper- and lower- body strength observed in the creatine group compared to the placebo group was probably due to higher quality training sessions.

Warber et al. (1998) randomly assigned 25 U.S. soldiers to either placebo or creatine (24 g/day for 5 days, 120 g total). Prior to and after supplementation, subjects performed a bench press protocol consisting of five sets of repetitions to fatigue with a resistance of 70% of 1-RM. Creatine supplementation resulted in a 14.4% increase in the total number of repetitions to fatigue. The authors concluded that creatine supplementation improves performance in a controlled strength test.

Mixed Ergogenic Effects   The following two studies have reported both ergogenic and nonergogenic effects of creatine supplementation on isotonic performance. Goldberg and Bechtel (1997) randomly assigned 34 male football and track athletes to either placebo or creatine (3 g/day for 14 days, 42 g total) groups in order to study the effects of low-dose supplementation on lower body strength and 1-RM bench press performance. During the study, subjects were concurrently engaged in off-season resistive training and were tested at baseline, 7 days, and 14 days of supplementation. The authors reported that creatine supplementation resulted in significant improvement in leg extension strength, but not in bench press performance.

Stout et al. (1999) reported contrasting results regarding the effects of two supplements that included creatine on bench press 1-RM in 24 football players. One supplement contained creatine monohydrate plus glucose; the other was Phosphagen HP™, containing creatine monohydrate plus sodium/potassium phosphates and taurine. The supplemented groups received the same amount of creatine monohydrate (21 g/day for 5 days, 105 g total). Subjects were randomly assigned to one of the two supplementation groups or to placebo (35 g glucose powder). Improvement in bench press 1-RM was significantly greater following Phosphagen HP™ supplementation (28.8 kg) compared to placebo (13.1 kg), with no difference in improvement between the creatine monohydrate supplementation (17.5 kg) and placebo groups. This study is somewhat difficult to interpret because of the discordant results obtained between treatments with the two creatine-containing supplements.

Studies Reporting No Ergogenic Effects   In addition to the studies of Goldberg and Bechtel (1997) and Stout et al. (1999), five other studies revealed no significant effect of creatine supplementation on isotonic exercise performance. Besides measuring isometric performance, Bermon et al. (1998) also measured isotonic strength (1-RM) and endurance (12-RM) for leg press, leg extension, and chest press before and after training in 32 elderly male and female subjects (67-80 years). Subjects were randomly assigned to one of four groups: sedentary-placebo; sedentary-creatine; training-placebo; and training-creatine. Supplementation consisted of an 8-week supplementation period. During the 8-week supplementation period (20 g/day for 5 d [100 g], followed by 3 g/d for 47 d [141 g, 241 g total], the training groups completed three sets of 8 repetitions at 80 percent of one-repetition maximum (1-RM) in leg press, leg extension, and chest press exercises 3 days/week. As was the case with isometric performance, there were no creatine, training, or interaction (supplementation by training) effects on isotonic strength or endurance for chest press, leg press, or leg extension force exercises. The authors concluded that creatine supplementation, either alone or in combination with training, did not improve isotonic performance in healthy elderly subjects.

Hamilton-Ward et al. (1997) randomly assigned 20 female athletes paired on body composition and age to either a placebo or creatine-supplementation (25 g/day for 7 days; 175 g total) group. Dependent variables included isotonic elbow flexion 1-RM and muscle fatigue during elbow flexion, measured as the number of repetitions at 70% of 1-RM. After creatine supplementation, the number of postsupplementation elbow flexion repetitions (15.0) was 16% greater than the number of presupplementation repetitions (12.9). However, this change was not statistically significant. It was concluded that creatine supplementation did not affect muscle strength or endurance.

Stevenson and Dudley (1998) randomly assigned 10 resistance-trained males to either a placebo or supplementation (20 g/day for 7 days, 140 g total) group to investigate the effects of creatine on knee extension 1-RM. There was no improvement in 1-RM performance following creatine supplementation. Subjects also completed five sets at 55% of knee extension 1-RM before and after creatine supplementation. There were no group differences, but a trend toward a significant group-by-time interaction ($p = 0.06$) was observed, with the creatine group performing 9.5% more repetitions after supplementation (pre- = 42 vs. post- = 46) compared to the placebo group (pre- = 42 vs. post- = 43). The authors suggested that the trend toward a significantly greater number of repetitions during multi-set resistive exercise may be explained either by the ergogenicity of creatine or by the neural adaptations to resistive exercise.

Syrotuik et al. (1998) studied the effects of creatine supplementation on a group of 21 untrained males who were participating in resistive-exercise training. Subjects were randomly assigned to either placebo or supplementation (20 g/day for 5 days, 100 g total) followed by a maintenance regimen (2 g/day for 32 days, ~64 g total). Isotonic strength was measured on the bench and inclined leg press (1-RM), with endurance measured by repetitions to fatigue at 50% of bench and inclined leg press 1-RM. Creatine supplementation failed to improve strength and endurance performance.

Finally, Wood et al. (1998) randomly assigned 44 weight-trained males to 42 days of either creatine (20 g/day for 5 days; 2 g/day for 37 days), placebo, or no supplementation. Prior to and after supplementation, bench press 1-RM was measured. Creatine supplementation had no effect on bench press 1-RM performance.

Effect of Different Forms of Creatine on Isotonic Performance   Several studies have compared the effect of different forms of creatine (e.g., powder vs. candy; creatine monohydrate vs. creatine phosphate) on isotonic performance. Crowder et al. (1998) compared the effects of two different forms of creatine on 1-RM for power clean, bench press, and squat in lightweight football players. Subjects were randomly assigned to one of the two groups and received supplementation in the form of either creatine powder or gum for three days. The daily dose was apparently 5 g/day for a total of 15 g, although this was unclear in the description of the supplementation regimen. Although improvement in isotonic strength was observed, the absence of a real control group makes it difficult to evaluate the ergogenic effect of this study.

Vukovich and Michaelis (1999) compared the effects of creatine powder (20 g/day for 5 days, 100 g total), creatine candy (20 g/day for 5 days, 100 g total) with those of powder placebo and candy placebo treatments on leg press 1-RM in 48 males. The initial supplementation regimen was followed by a maintenance regimen of 10 g/day for 16 days (160 g total). The increases in leg press 1-RM observed after creatine powder supplementation (63.1 kg) and creatine candy (52.9 kg) were greater than the increases observed for powder placebo (32.3 kg) and candy placebo (30.6 kg).

Peeters et al. (1999) compared the effects of creatine phosphate and creatine monohydrate supplementation on isotonic strength and endurance as measured by bench and leg press 1-RM and repetitions to exhaustion. Thirty-nine strength-trained males were randomly assigned to either one of two supplementation or placebo groups. Initial supplementation (20 g/day for 3 days, 60 g total) was provided, followed by an additional 10 g/day for 6 weeks (420 g total). After 3 weeks of creatine monohydrate supplementation, bench press 1-RM improved by 9.6%. An increase in bench press 1-RM was also observed following 3 weeks of creatine phosphate supplementation. Leg press 1-RM and repetitions to fatigue were not improved at 3 weeks by either creatine phosphate or monohydrate supplementation. At 6 weeks, strength performance was constant or improved for both supplementation groups compared to the placebo group.

Summary   Improvement in performance of both single-effort isotonic strength (Becque et al. 1997; Crowder et al. 1998; Earnest et al. 1995; Goldberg and Bechtel, 1997; Knehans et al. 1998; Kreider et al. 1998b; Larson et al. 1998; Noonan et al. 1998b; Pearson et al. 1998; Peeters et al. 1999; Stone et al. 1999; Stout et al. 1999) and repetitive endurance (Kelly and Jenkins 1998; Volek et al. 1997a; Vukovich and Michaelis 1999; Warber et al. 1998) tasks has been reported following creatine supplementation. Populations in which ergogenic effects have been observed are predominantly 20-30-year-old males described as either trained individuals (Becque et al. 1997; Earnest et al. 1995; Kelly and Jenkins 1998; Peeters et al. 1999; Volek et al. 1997a, 1997b; Warber et al. 1998) or elite athletes (Crowder et al. 1998; Knehans et al. 1998; Kreider et al. 1998b; Pearson et al. 1998; Stone et al. 1999). The study of Larson et al. (1998) is the only one reporting an ergogenic effect in females. Eight studies employed longer supplementation regimens of 4-5 weeks (Kelly and Jenkins 1998; Kreider et al. 1998b; Stone et al. 1999), 6-8 weeks (Knehans et al. 1998; Noonan et al. 1998b; Pearson et al. 1998; Peeters et al. 1999; Wood et al. 1998), and 10-13 weeks (Larson et al. 1998). Five of these studies (Knehans et al. 1998; Noonan et al. 1998b; Pearson et al. 1998; Peeters et al. 1999; Volek et al. 1999) presented evidence of improvement in performance past 4 weeks. The available literature supports the conclusion that in some individuals, creatine supplementation may improve performance in such isotonic tasks as 1-RM and number of repetitions to fatigue.

Of 23 studies that have evaluated the effect of creatine supplementation on isotonic strength/endurance, 17 showed improvements (15% for 11 of the 16 studies; median = 9%) in various measures of isotonic strength and endurance following creatine supplementation. The available data support the conclusion that creatine supplementation may improve performance in such isotonic resistance tasks as 1-RM and number of repetitions to fatigue. Eight studies showed no beneficial effect after creatine supplementation. Of these eight studies, two reported both ergogenic and negative effects, and none showed an ergolytic effect.

Isokinetic Force Production

Studies of creatine supplementation and isokinetic torque/force production are presented in table 5.3. Of the 14 studies discussed in this section, 7 show improvement (mean 14% improvement; median = 8%) following creatine supplementation. In the remaining studies there was no effect of creatine supplementation on isokinetic force production. Two studies (Grindstaff et al. 1995; Vandenberghe et al. 1997a) reported both ergogenic and nonergogenic results. No study has shown an ergolytic effect.

Studies Reporting Ergogenic Effects   Greenhaff et al. (1993b) investigated the influence of creatine monohydrate supplementation on muscle torque during repeated bouts of maximal voluntary exercise in 12 physically active, but not highly trained, subjects randomly assigned to placebo or supplementation (20 g/day for 5 days, 100 g total). Subjects completed five bouts of 30 maximal voluntary isokinetic contractions, interspersed with recovery periods of 1 min, before and after supplementation. The contractions were partitioned into three segments of contractions (contractions 1-10, 11-20, and 21-30). No difference was seen in muscle torque production during exercise before and after placebo ingestion. However, muscle peak torque production after creatine supplementation was greater in all subjects during the final 10 contractions of exercise bout 1, throughout the whole of exercise bouts 2, 3, and 4, and during contractions 11-20 of the final exercise bout. The authors concluded that creatine supplementation may accelerate skeletal muscle PCr resynthesis, and that the increased availability of PCr would better maintain the required rate of ATP demand during muscle contraction.

Grindstaff et al. (1995) assigned 18 resistance-trained males to either a placebo or acute supplementation (20 g/day for 7 days, 140 g total) group. Subjects performed five sets of 15 maximal-effort isokinetic bench press and squat repetitions. A significant 6% increase was observed in bench press peak power after supplementation.

Johnson et al. (1997) measured concentric and eccentric power and work in a bilateral knee extensor test to exhaustion prior to and after creatine supplementation (20 g/day for 6 days, 120 g total) in 18 males and females who were randomly assigned to either a placebo or creatine group. After creatine supplementation, subjects increased concentric and eccentric power by 6% and 9%, respectively. Increases of 25% and 15% were also reported for concentric and eccentric work for the right leg. The authors concluded that creatine supplementation was effective in improving muscular isokinetic power and work.

Using a crossover design, Vandenberghe et al. (1996a) measured isokinetic torque production in nine healthy, sedentary males before and after creatine supplementation (40 g/day for 6 days, 240 g total). Muscle [PCr]/[ß-ATP] ratio increased as measured by ^{31}P-MRS. Subjects performed maximal voluntary contractions in three interval series of 3 sets $\times$ 30, 4 sets $\times$ 20, and 5 sets $\times$ 10 contractions separated by 2 min rest. Isokinetic torque production increased by 10-23% after creatine supplementation, with the most noticeable improvement

Table 5.3 Effect of Creatine Supplementation on High-Intensity, Short-Duration ($\leq$ 30 sec) Single or Repetitive Isokinetic (IK) Resistive Exercise Performance Tasks Involving the Adenosine Triphosphate-Phosphocreatine (ATP-PCr) Energy System. Studies Are Arranged According to Ergogenic Effects.

Investigator	Year	Population	N	Gender	Design	Initial CM dose g × d = dose			Mode	Ergogenic effect?	%Δ	Comments
Greenhaff et al.	1993b	Physically active	12	M/F	RDBPC	20	5	100	30 reps × 5 sets	Y	6.8	Greater absolute leg torque and attenuated decline in torque after CM supplementation.
Grindstaff et al.	1995	Resistance trained	18	M	RDBPC	20	7	140	5 × 15 maximal bench and squat	Y	6	Increase in bench press peak power.
Johnson et al.	1997	Volunteers	18	M/F	RDBPC	20	6	120	Concentric and eccentric power and work of knee extensors	Y	6	Respectfully increases of 6% and 9% for concentric and eccentric power, and 25% and 15% for concentric and eccentric work.
Vandenberghe et al.	1997a	Healthy, sedentary	19	F	RDBPC	20 5	4 70	80 350	Elbow flexion power (70% 1-RM 5 × 30 reps)	Y	25	Arm flexion torque was increased in 5th set. CM + resistance training increased

(continued)

Table 5.3 (continued)

Investigator	Year	Population	N	Gender	Design	Initial CM dose g × d = dose			Mode	Ergogenic effect?	%Δ	Comments
Vandenberghe et al. (cont.)												training volume, reduced fatigue, and accelerated muscle hypertrophy after 10 weeks.
Vandenberghe et al.	1999	Healthy volunteers	9	M	RDBPC	25	5	125	5 × 30 max voluntary contractions with 2 min rest	Y	5-13	Increased performance similar at both 2 days and 5 days of supplementation.
Vandenberghe et al.	1996a	Healthy	9	M	RDBPCX	40	6	240	3 × 30 reps/ 4 × 20 reps/ 5 × 10 reps, at 180°/sec	Y	23	Increase in torque of 10-23%.
Ziegenfuss et al.	1998a	Omnivorous	16	M	RDBPC	25	5	125	6 sets at 90°/sec; 1 set at 180°/sec; knee extension	Y	7.4	Tested at baseline, 7, 14, 21, 28 d. Increases were retained at 28 d.
Almada et al.	1995	Resistance trained	18	M	RDBPC	20	28	560	5 × 15 maximal bench and squat	N		

Study	Year	Subjects	Age	Sex	Design				Measure	Result
Brees	1994	Vegans vs. meat-eaters	20	F	RDBPCX	25	5	125	Leg extension power (4 × 15 max)	N
Gilliam et al.	1998	Active, untrained	23	M	RDBPC	20	5	100	Right leg extension at 180°/sec; 5 sets × 30	N
Grindstaff et al.	1995	Resistance trained	18	M	RDBPC	20	7	140	5 × 15 maximal bench and squat	N
Hamilton-Ward et al.	1997	Athletes	20	F	RDBPC	25	7	175	Elbow flexion torque	N
Kreider et al.	1995	Resistance trained	18	M	RDBPC	13.5	7	95	Concentric 5 × 15 max bench	N
Kreider et al.	1996	Football players	43	M	RDBPC	20 25.5	35 35	700 or 892	1-RM concentric bench press at 0.25, 0.99, and 1.74 m/sec; 5 × 15 sec max effort bench reps at 0.25 m/sec with 60 sec rest	N

(continued)

Table 5.3 *(continued)*

Investigator	Year	Population	N	Gender	Design	Initial CM dose g × d = dose			Mode	Ergogenic effect? %Δ	Comments
Rawson et al.	1998	Older	16	M	RDBPC	20	5	100	Knee extensions, 3 × 30 reps at 180°/sec	N	
Vandenberghe	1997a	Healthy, sedentary	19	F	RDBPC	20	4	80	Elbow flexion power at 70% 1-RM; 5 × 30	N	

CM = creatine monohydrate; PL = placebo; RDBPC = Randomized, double-blind, placebo control
RDBPCX = Randomized, double-blind, placebo control, crossover

observed immediately after the 2 min rest between sets. This observation supports the hypothesis of enhanced postexercise ATP resynthesis due to increased [PCr] after supplementation (Casey et al. 1996; Greenhaff et al. 1993a, 1994a).

Using a similar design, Vandenberghe et al. (1997b) also investigated the effects of creatine (25 g/day for 5 days, 125 g total), caffeine plus creatine (2 × 2.5 mg/kg body mass/day) and placebo on isokinetic force production (5 × 30 knee extension MVC with a 2 min rest interval between sets) in nine males. Treatments were administered in a counterbalanced manner and separated by a 5 week washout period. Muscle [creatine], measured by ^{31}P-MRS, was similarly increased (8-15%) two and five days following both creatine and caffeine plus creatine treatments. There was evidence of reduced PCr resynthesis following the ingestion of the supplement containing caffeine plus creatine. Compared to placebo, increased torque production in successive knee extension bouts, measured in Newton meters, was observed both two days (5-8%) and five days (7-13%) following creatine ingestion. This ergogenic effect was not observed following the creatine plus caffeine supplementation. The authors concluded that two days of creatine supplementation increased muscle [PCr] and improved isokinetic force production to the same extent as five days of supplementation. Furthermore, muscle PCr resynthesis during intermittent exercise was impaired by the combination of caffeine and creatine. An expanded discussion of this study, with the caffeine data removed, has been published elsewhere (Vandenberghe et al. 1999).

In another study, Vandenberghe et al. (1997a) randomly assigned 19 healthy, sedentary females to either a placebo or high-dose creatine-supplementation phase (20 g/day for 4 days, 80 g total) followed by a low-dose supplementation phase (5 g/day for 10 weeks, 350 g total). Muscle [PCr]/[ß-ATP] ratio, measured by ^{31}P-MRS, was increased following the high-dose phase, but elbow flexion power output at 70% 1-RM was unchanged. Muscle [PCr]/[ß-ATP] ratio remained elevated throughout the low-dose phase, and elbow flexion power output increased in the creatine group after this phase. The authors concluded that creatine supplementation increased training volume, reduced fatigue, and accelerated muscle hypertrophy.

Ziegenfuss et al. (1998a) randomly assigned 16 omnivorous males to either placebo or supplementation (350 mg/kg body mass [~25 g/day] for 5 days, 125 g total) to examine the prolonged effects of acute creatine supplementation. Subjects performed one set of knee extension exercise at 90°/sec and one set at 180°/sec prior to, immediately after, and 7, 14, and 21 days after cessation of supplementation. Knee extension torque increased by 7.4%. An interesting aspect of this study was that this improvement was retained 21 days after the end of supplementation.

Studies Reporting No Ergogenic Effects   The studies discussed in the remainder of this section do not support the ergogenicity of creatine on isokinetic force production. Almada et al. (1995) studied the effects of a longer supplementation regimen (20 g/day for 28 days, 560 g total) on power production in five sets of 15 maximal isokinetic bench press and squat repetitions. Eighteen resistance-trained males were randomly assigned to either a placebo or supplementation group. There was no improvement in bench press or squat power after supplementation.

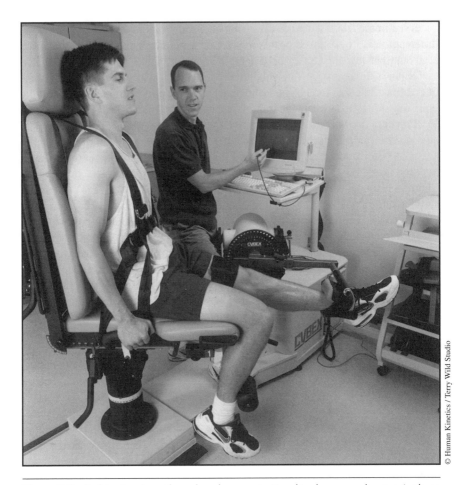

© Human Kinetics / Terry Wild Studio

Figure 5.3 Isokinetic strength and endurance testing has been used extensively to evaluate the ergogenic effects of creatine.

Brees et al. (1994) compared the effects of creatine supplementation on female vegetarians and meat-eaters. Subjects received both placebo and acute supplementation (25 g/day for 5 days, 125 g total) in a counterbalanced manner, with treatments separated by a 3-week washout period. The exercise protocol consisted of four sets of 15 maximal isokinetic leg extensions for measurement of concentric and eccentric power. Pooled group analysis of data revealed a significant 5.7% increase in mean power output following creatine supplementation compared to presupplementation. It should also be noted that a 4.7% improvement was observed after the placebo treatment. Thus, there was no difference between dietary groups in the response to creatine supplementation. However, it is unclear whether the authors counterbalanced treatment order within dietary groups. If not, the short washout period may be a potential confounding influence on the results of this study.

Gilliam et al. (1998) randomly assigned 23 active, untrained males to either placebo or acute supplementation (20 g/day for 5 days, 100 g total). Subjects were measured before and after supplementation on an isokinetic exercise protocol consisting of five sets of 30 right leg extension repetitions performed at 180°/sec. There was no improvement in peak torque, either within or between groups, after creatine supplementation.

In a study discussed earlier in this section, Grindstaff et al. (1995) randomly assigned 18 resistance-trained males to either placebo or creatine supplementation (20 g/day for 7 days, 140 g total) groups. Isokinetic bench press and squat performance (5 sets × 15 maximal-effort repetitions) were measured prior to and after supplementation. Although a 6% increase in bench press peak power was observed after creatine supplementation, there was no improvement in absolute or relative bench press force, average force, average power loss, or squat performance.

Hamilton-Ward et al. (1997) investigated the effects of acute supplementation (25 g/day for 7 days, 175 g total) on peak shoulder internal rotation velocity (degrees/sec), as well as concentric and eccentric elbow torque, in 20 female athletes. Although postsupplementation elbow flexion torque improved by 8.9% compared to the presupplementation value, this increase was not significant. The authors concluded that isokinetic performance remained unchanged following creatine supplementation.

Using 18 resistance-trained males as subjects, Kreider et al. (1995) examined the effects of a supplement that included creatine (13.5 g/day for 7 days, 94.5 g total), taurine, ribonucleic acid, carbohydrate, and protein on concentric bench press and squat performance. Subjects were randomly assigned to either a placebo or supplement group. The exercise protocol consisted of five sets of 15 maximal concentric bench press repetitions performed at a velocity of 0.25 m/sec with 60 sec rest between sets. The authors reported that this supplement had no significant effect on slow-velocity concentric bench press performance.

In another study, Kreider et al. (1996a) studied the effects of two creatine supplements (Phosphagain™ with 20 g creatine/day for 35 days, 700 g total; and Phosphagain™ with 25.5 g creatine/day for 35 days, 893 g total) and placebo on isokinetic bench press performance in 43 college football players. Prior to and after supplementation, subjects completed 1-RM concentric-only bench press at 0.25, 0.99, and 1.74 m/sec. They also completed 5 × 15 maximal-effort repetitions at 0.25 m/sec with a 60 sec rest interval between sets. Comparison of both supplementation groups to placebo revealed a trend toward greater gains in total work performed at 0.99 m/sec after supplementation (p = 0.053). No other effects of creatine supplementation on isokinetic strength or endurance were observed.

The effects of creatine supplementation on an older population was studied by Rawson et al. (1998), who randomly assigned 16 males ranging in age from 60 to 78 years to either a placebo or acute supplementation (20 g/day for 5 days, 100 g total) group. Subjects completed three sets of 30 isokinetic knee extension repetitions performed at 180°/sec. The dependent variable was total peak torque generated during each bout of exercise. Although a significant group-by-trial interaction was observed, it was apparently the result of decreased performance in the placebo group rather than improved performance in the creatine group. The authors concluded that the small increases in isokinetic torque observed in older males following creatine supplementation were not significant.

As the initial phase of their study of chronic supplementation during resistance training, Vandenberghe et al. (1997a) measured elbow flexion power in five sets of 30 repetitions performed at 70% of 1-RM in 19 healthy, sedentary females who were assigned to either placebo or short-term "high-dose" supplementation (20 g/day for 4 days, 80 g total). Both muscle [PCr] and the [PCr]/[ß-ATP] ratio increased by 6% after the high-dose phase as measured by ^{31}P-MRS. Although the authors reported slight improvement in torque following the high-dose phase, the improvement was not significant.

Summary   Most of the studies supporting the ergogenicity of creatine on isokinetic performance show improvements in torque and/or force production during repetitive exercise following short-term ($\leq$ 7 days) (Brees et al. 1994; Greenhaff et al. 1993b; Grindstaff et al. 1995; Johnson et al. 1997; Vandenberghe et al. 1996a; 1997b; Ziegenfuss et al. 1998a) or chronic (Vandenberghe et al. 1997a) supplementation. Although the results are divergent with regard to the ergogenicity of creatine, the available evidence suggests that supplementation may improve isokinetic torque force production and attenuate the decline in power during repetitive isokinetic exercise in a laboratory setting.

Of 14 studies that have evaluated the effect of creatine supplementation on isokinetic strength/endurance, 7 showed improvement (mean = 14%; median = 8%) after creatine supplementation. The remaining studies show no effect of creatine supplementation on isokinetic force production, and no study has shown an ergolytic effect. Most of the studies supporting the ergogenicity of creatine on isokinetic performance show improvements in torque and/or force production during repetitive exercise following acute supplementation.

Cycle Ergometer Performance

Various short-term, high-intensity cycle ergometer protocols have been used to investigate the possible ergogenic effect of creatine supplementation, with time frames ranging from 6 to 30 sec. The studies in this section are stratified and discussed in order according to (1) ergogenic result (significant vs. nonsignificant) and (2) type of cycle ergometer task (repetitive vs. single bout). Table 5.4 provides a summary of the studies discussed in this section.

Studies Reporting Ergogenic Effects on Repetitive Cycle Ergometer Protocols   Here we describe 18 studies that show a mean of 16% improvement (median = 7%) in performance in various repetitive cycle ergometer tasks.

Balsom et al. (1993a) randomly assigned 16 highly motivated, well-trained male physical education students to either a placebo or creatine-supplementation (25 g/day) group and had them undergo two intermittent high-intensity cycle ergometer exercise protocols before and after 6 days of supplementation. The total creatine ingested was 150 g. The first exercise protocol involved 10 bouts × 6 sec isokinetic cycling at 130 rev/min (~820 W) interspersed with 30 sec of passive rest. The second protocol was designed to induce fatigue so that subjects would be unable to maintain force output throughout each 6 sec period over the 10 exercise bouts (10 × 6 sec at 140 rev/min [~880 W]). The work output of each 6 sec bout was partitioned into three intervals (0-2 sec, 2-4 sec, and 4-6 sec). Theoretically, creatine supplementation would be most beneficial in the latter intervals, that is, 4-6 sec. The authors noted that significant differences in this time frame between the groups began after the 7th bout, with the creatine group experiencing a significantly lower decrease in performance compared to the placebo group. Examination of their data plots also indicated that although the performance of the placebo group declined from bout 1 through bout 3, the performance of the creatine group actually increased during these first 3 bouts. However, the differences became increasingly greater after trial 4 and became statistically significant after trial 7.

In a later study, Balsom et al. (1995) recruited seven highly motivated, physically active male subjects to perform repeated bouts of fixed-intensity cycle ergometer exercise (5 × 6 sec with 30 sec recovery periods), followed by a maximal 10 sec bout to determine maximal power output, before and after creatine supplementation (20 g/day for 6 days, 120 g total). Supplementation resulted in an increase in muscle [PCr] as measured by needle biopsy. Following supplementation, subjects were able to maintain power output, as demonstrated by an attenuated rate of decline in pedal frequency at the end of the 10 sec bout. The authors concluded that creatine supplementation enhanced resistance to fatigue.

Birch et al. (1994) randomly assigned 14 healthy, but not highly trained, male subjects to either a creatine or placebo group to investigate 3 × 30 sec power and work performance bouts. The bouts were performed at 80 rev/min with 4 min rest. Subjects in the creatine group received the standard short-term loading regimen (20 g/day for 5 days, 100 g total creatine) with no additional supplementation. Significant increases in peak power output (8% for the first bout), mean power output (6% for the first two bouts), and total work (6% for the first two bouts) were observed in the creatine group. The authors concluded that whole-body performance can be improved in the first two of three maximal 30 sec bouts.

Casey et al. (1996) investigated the effect of acute supplementation (20 g/day for 5 days, 100 g total creatine) on isokinetic cycle performance (2 × 30 sec at 80 rev/min with 4 min passive rest) in nine healthy males. Muscle creatine uptake was measured by needle biopsy. Creatine supplementation resulted in a significant 19% increase in muscle [TCr]. Following supplementation, significant increases in total work production (joule/kg body mass) were reported for bout 1 (4.2%) and bout 2 (4.4%). The authors reported the increases in peak and total work to be positively correlated with the increases in muscle [TCr], specifically in type II fibers.

Table 5.4 Effect of Creatine Supplementation on High-Intensity, Short-Duration ($\leq$ 30 sec) Single or Repetitive Cycle Ergometer (CE) Performance Tasks Involving the Adenosine Triphosphate-Phosphocreatine (ATP-PCr) Energy System. Studies Are Arranged According to Ergogenic Effects.

Investigator	Year	Population	N	Gender	Design	Initial CM dose g × d = dose			Mode	Ergogenic effect?	%Δ	Comments
Balsom et al.	1995	Physically active	7	M	SGRM	20	6	120	5 × 6 sec; 1 × 10 sec	Y	5	Increased power during 10 sec trial.
Balsom et al.	1993a	Active / well trained	16	M	RDBPC	25	6	150	10 × 6 sec 130 rev/min (~820 W)	Y	N/A	
									10 × 6 sec 140 rev/min (~880 W)			Attenuated decline in power across the 10 trials.
Birch et al.	1994	Healthy, not highly trained	14	M	RDBPC	20	5	100	30 × 30 sec	Y	10.5	Increase in peak and mean power and work for bouts 1 and 2.
Casey et al.	1996	Healthy	9	M	SGRM	20	5	100	2 × 30 sec isokinetic cycling	Y	4	Increase in peak power and total work for bout 2.
Dawson et al.	1995	Healthy active	22	M	RDBPC	20	5	100	6 × 6 sec	Y	4.6	Increase in peak power and total work.
Earnest et al.	1995	Healthy	24	M/F	RDBPC	20	5	100	Wingate (× 2)	Y	12.9	Increase in power observed following

(continued)

												Findings
												initial loading. No effects of acute CM ingestion over initial loading regimen.
Earnest et al.	1995	Weight trained	8	M	RDBPC	20	14	280	Wingate (× 3)	Y	18	Increase in total work for all tests.
Greenhaff et al.	1994b	Healthy recreational athletes	6	M	SGRM	20	5	100	Isokinetic cycling (2 × 30 sec at 80 rev/min)	Y	4.9	Increase in total work for 2nd bout with 50% reduction in loss of ATP and 19.4% increase in muscle [TCr].
Jones et al.	1998	Elite ice hockey players	16	M	RDBPC	20 / 10	5 / 70	100 / 700	5 × 15 sec "all-out" sprints	Y	20.7	Increase in mean work and peak power following initial loading, with no further improvement with maintenance dose.
Kamber et al.	1999	Well-trained sports students	10	M	RDBPCX	20	5	100	10 × 6-sec maximal sprints (rev/min) with 30 sec rest	Y	3.5	Increase in mean performance for all 10 sprints following creatine supplementation compared to placebo

Table 5.4 (continued)

Investigator	Year	Population	N	Gender	Design	Initial CM dose g × d = dose			Mode	Ergogenic effect?	%Δ	Comments
Kamber (cont.)												(0.7%). Higher rev/min in the last 2 sec of sprints 4-10 following creatine supplementation.
Kirksey et al.	1997	Track and field athletes	36	M/F	RDBPC	20	42	840	Wingate (× 5)	Y	13	Increase in mean peak power for all tests.
Kreider et al.	1998b	Football players	25	M	RDBPC	15.75	28	441	12 × 6 sec sprints	Y	N/A	Total sprint work was increased following CM.
Kreider et al.	1998a	Untrained/trained	50	M/F	RDBPC	16.5 15.75	14	231 220.5	6 × 6 sec sprints	Y	N/A	Comparison of CM and Phosphagain HP™. Both improved average work for each sprint, with no difference between treatments.
Prevost et al.	1997	Physically active college students	18	M/F	RSBPC	19	5	94	Time to exhaustion (150% VO_{2max})	Y	61	30 sec work/60 sec rest intermittent protocol.

Author	Year	Subjects	N	Sex	Design				Test		Y/N		Results
									30 sec/ 60 sec rest				
									Time to exhaustion (150% VO_{2max}) 20 sec/ 40 sec rest		Y	62	20 sec work/ 40 sec rest intermittent protocol.
									Time to exhaustion (150% VO_{2max}) 10 sec/ 20 sec rest		Y	100	10 sec work/ 20 sec rest intermittent protocol.
Schneider et al.	1997	Untrained	9	M	SBPC	25	7	175	5 × 15 sec		Y	6.5	Increase in total work (p = 0.10).
Theodoru et al.	1998	Physical education students	20	M	RDBPC	25	4	100	Wingate test (× 3)		Y	5.5	Compared to baseline, improvement in mean power overall, 5.1% improvement for 2nd test, 8.5% improvement for 3rd test.
						25	4	100	Wingate test (× 3)		Y	2.7	Ingestion of creatine with 500 ml CHO drink. No difference in mean power

(continued)

Table 5.4 *(continued)*

Investigator	Year	Population	N	Gender	Design	Initial CM dose g × d = dose			Mode	Ergogenic effect?	%Δ	Comments
Theodoru et al. *(cont.)*												overall, but 6.7% improvement for 3rd test.
Vukovich and Michaelis	1999	Resistance trained	48	M	RDBPC	20 10	5 16	100 160	5 × 10 sec sprints at 5 J/kg/rev	Y	N/A	Improved performance for groups ingesting creatine powder or candy compared to placebo.
Ziegenfuss et al.	1997	High power	33	M/F	RDBPC	20	3	60	6 × 10 sec	Y	N/A	Increase in total work in sprint 1; increase in peak power sprints 2-6.
Barnett et al.	1996	Recreationally active	17	M	RSBPC	20	4	80	7 × 10 sec sprints	N		
Burke et al.	1996	Elite swimmers	32	M/F	RDBPC	20	5	100	2 × 10 sec sprints	N		
Chetlin et al.	1998	Resistance trained	33	M	RDBPC	20	10	200	Wingate test	N		
Cooke and Barnes	1997	Healthy active	80	M	RDBPC	20	5	100	2 maximal sprints/ recovery	N		

Reference	Year	Subjects	N	Sex	Design				Protocol	
Cooke et al.	1995	Untrained	12	M	RDBPC	20	5	100	2 × 15 sec	N
Dawson et al.	1995	Healthy active	18	M	RDBPC	20	5	100	1 × 10 sec	N
Gonzalez de Suso et al.	1995	Trained	19	M/F	RDBPCX	21	14	294	7 × 7 sec	N
Ledford and Branch	1999	Trained	9	F	RDBPCX	20	5	100	Wingate (× 3)	N
Odland et al.	1997	Physically active	9	M	SGRM	20	3	60	Wingate	N
Ruden et al.	1996	College aged	9	M/F	SGRM	20	4	80	Wingate	N
Snow et al.	1998	Active untrained	8	M	RDBPCX	30	5	150	20 sec single sprint	N
Stone et al.	1999	Football players	42	M	RDBPC	20	35	700	15 × 5 sec sprints with 1 min rest	N
			8			35	280			

CM = creatine monohydrate   CHO = carbohydrate   RDBPC = Randomized, double-blind, placebo control
RDBPCX = Randomized, double-blind, placebo control, crossover   RSBPC = Randomized, single-blind, placebo control
SGPC = single group, placebo control   SGRM = single group, repeated measures

They concluded that the improvements in work output were related to enhanced ATP resynthesis secondary to increased [PCr] in type II fibers.

Dawson et al. (1995) measured sprint performance (6 bouts $\times$ 6 sec with a 24 sec recovery period between bouts) in 22 subjects who were randomly assigned to either a placebo or short-term supplementation (20 g/day for 5 days, 100 g total) group. Increases in peak power output (4.6%) and total work (4.6%) were observed in the creatine group after supplementation. The creatine group also completed more work in sprint 1 (in isolation) compared to the placebo group.

Earnest et al. (1995) used three Wingate tests (30 sec) interspersed with a 5 min rest as their test protocol to study the effect of creatine monohydrate (20 g/day for 14 days, 280 g total) ingestion on peak anaerobic power (highest power output in a 5 sec period) and capacity (total work in 30 sec). Eight weight-trained males were matched according to mean anaerobic capacity and assigned to either a placebo or supplementation group. Although there were no significant differences between the groups with regard to peak anaerobic power, the creatine group experienced a significant improvement in total work capacity in all three Wingate tests (13%, 18%, and 18%), while the placebo group experienced no changes.

Subsequent to the study just cited, Earnest et al. (1998) provided 24 subjects with short-term creatine supplementation (20 g/day for 5 days, 100 g total). The unique aspect of this study was investigation of the effect of ingestion of a single creatine dose (10 g ingested 1 h prior to exercise) on cycle ergometer performance after this initial loading phase. Subjects received either 10 g of creatine, 80 g of dextrose, or 10 g of creatine plus 80 g of dextrose. The test protocol consisted of two Wingate tests separated by a 5 min rest interval. A within-group 13% increase in power was observed after the initial 5-day loading regimen. However, the single 10 g dose was ineffective in eliciting further improvement over that observed following the initial loading regimen.

In a single group, ordered, repeated-measures design, Greenhaff et al. (1994b) investigated the effect of creatine supplementation (20 g/day for 5 days, 100 g total) on isokinetic cycle ergometer exercise (2 bouts $\times$ 30 sec at 80 rev/min with 4 min rest interval) in six healthy male subjects. Creatine ingestion resulted in a 19% increase in muscle [TCr], measured by needle biopsy, as well as a significant increase in total work in the second bout. The authors reported a 50% reduction in ATP loss in the second exercise bout after supplementation, despite a 4.9% increase in work performance, suggesting that a possible consequence of increased [TCr] ([PCr]+[creatine]) is an attenuation of ATP degradation during intense work.

Jones et al. (1998) randomly assigned 16 NCAA Division I ice hockey players to either a placebo or creatine-supplementation (20 g/day for 5 days, 100 g total) group. The initial loading phase was followed by a maintenance phase (10 g/day for 10 weeks, 700 g total). The exercise protocol consisted of 5 $\times$ 15 sec "all-out" cycle ergometer sprints using a resistance of 0.075 kg per kg body mass. Subjects were tested at baseline, 10 days, and 10 weeks. Improvements in mean work (21%) and peak power were noted at 10 days compared to baseline. However, maintenance supplementation failed to elicit further improvement.

Kamber et al. (1999) employed a protocol similar to that reported by Balsom et al. (1993A) to investigate the effects of creatine supplementation (20 g/d for 5 days, 100 g total) compared to placebo on high-intensity sprint cycle ergometer performance (6×10 sec sprints with a 30 sec rest interval). Ten well-trained sport students received both creatine and placebo treatments in a crossover manner, with counterbalanced treatment order and a mean washout of 61 days. Following creatine supplementation, mean sprint performance (rev/min) was increased by 3.5% compared to no change following the placebo treatment. The ergogenic effect was most apparent in the last two sec (i.e. 4-6 sec) of the last six sprint bouts (i.e. bouts 4-10). No ergogenic effect was observed in the first two sec (0-2 sec) for any sprint. These results suggest that the ergogenic effects of creatine supplementation are more apparent in the latter seconds of repetitive, high-intensity, short-duration sprint cycle ergometry.

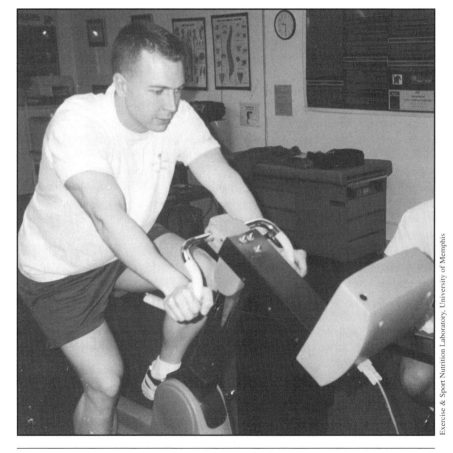

Exercise & Sport Nutrition Laboratory, University of Memphis

Figure 5.4 Various cycle ergometer exercise protocols, ranging from 6-30 sec, have been used extensively to study the effects of creatine on high power.

Kirksey et al. (1997) randomly assigned 36 male and female track and field athletes to either a placebo or supplementation (0.3 g/kg body mass per day [~20 g/day] for 6 weeks, 840 g total) group. Cycle ergometer performance (5×10 sec with 1 min recovery) was measured prior to and after supplementation. A significant group-by-trial interaction in mean peak power was observed across all five Wingate trials with a 13% increase in the creatine group as compared to a 5% increase in the placebo group. The authors concluded that creatine supplementation favorably increased power output in male and female track and field athletes.

Using a subject pool of 50 trained and untrained males and females, Kreider et al. (1997a) studied the effects of acute creatine monohydrate supplementation (16.5 g/day for 14 days, 238 g total) and Phosphagain HP™ supplementation (15.75 g creatine monohydrate/day for 14 days, 220.5 g total) or placebo on cycle ergometer performance. The exercise protocol was 6×6 sec sprints with 30 sec rest between bouts. Compared to the placebo group, both creatine monohydrate and Phosphagain HP™ groups improved average work per sprint. There were no differences between supplemented groups.

Kreider et al. (1998b) employed a similar protocol in a later study of 25 NCAA Division IA football players. Subjects were matched on body mass and assigned to 28 days of either a placebo or Phosphagain HP™ (15.75 g creatine monohydrate/day, 441 g total) supplementation. The cycle ergometer protocol consisted of 12×6 sec sprints with 30 sec rest. An increase in total work accomplished for the first five sprints was observed after creatine monohydrate supplementation.

Prevost et al. (1997) randomly assigned 18 college-aged, physically active males and females to placebo or creatine-supplementation groups. The initial creatine-supplementation regimen consisted of 18.75 g/day for 5 days (94 g total); subjects then received a maintenance dose of 2.25 g/day for 6 days (14 g total). Subjects were administered three different cycle ergometer intermittent-interval training regimens, each with a work component of less than 30 sec at 150% of $\dot{V}O_{2max}$. Creatine supplementation increased time to exhaustion by 61% for 30 sec work/60 sec rest, 62% for 20 sec work/40 sec rest, and 100% for 10 sec work/20 sec rest regimens. The authors concluded that the ability to maintain high-intensity, intermittent exercise is enhanced by creatine supplementation.

Using a single-blind design, Schneider et al. (1997) randomly assigned nine untrained males to a placebo or acute supplementation (25 g/day for 7 days, 175 g total) group. Total work performed in 5×15 sec cycle ergometer bouts was measured prior to and after supplementation. These investigators reported that creatine ingestion resulted in a significant ($p = 0.10$) 6.5% increase in total work (kJ) compared to the placebo treatment, suggesting that creatine supplementation may increase the rate of ATP resynthesis in untrained subjects. The authors concluded that creatine supplementation increased the capacity to maintain high-intensity, intermittent work.

Theodoru et al. (1998) examined the effects of creatine supplementation (25 g/day for 4 days, 100 g total), the same dose of creatine plus 500 ml carbohydrate solution, or placebo on three repetitions of the Wingate test performance. Twenty male physical education students were randomly assigned to one of the three groups. Improved mean power (5.5%) compared to baseline was observed over the three tests in the creatine group after supplementation with most of the improvement occurring in the second and third tests. Although the creatine plus carbohydrate group significantly improved performance by 6.7% in the third test, the overall 2.7% increase in mean power was not significant for the three tests.

Finally, Ziegenfuss et al. (1997) examined the effects of short-term supplementation (0.35 g/kg fat-free mass/day [~20 g/day] for 3 days, 60 g total) vs. placebo on performance in 33 male and female "high-power" subjects. The exercise protocol consisted of 6 × 10 sec cycle sprints. Muscle creatine was not measured. After supplementation, the authors observed increased (p = 0.10) total work capacity in the first sprint, with increased peak power in the last five sprints.

Effect of Different Forms of Creatine on Cycle Ergometer Performance   The primary focus of a study by Vukovich and Michaelis (1999) was to compare the effects of different creatine forms. Forty-eight males were randomly assigned to one of four groups: creatine powder or creatine candy supplementation groups (20 g/day for 5 days [100 g total] followed by 10 g/day for 16 days [160 g total]), or powder placebo or candy placebo groups. Subjects completed 5 × 10-sec sprints at 5 J/rev per kg body mass prior to and following the supplementation. The authors report that compared to the placebo groups, creatine supplementation improved cycle ergometer performance.

Studies Reporting No Ergogenic Effects on Repetitive Cycle Ergometer Protocols   In this section we describe seven studies that do not support the ergogenicity of creatine supplementation.

Barnett et al. (1996) employed a single-blind design to study the effects of acute supplementation (20 g/day for 4 days, 80 g total) on multiple sprint performance (7 × 10 sec) in 17 recreationally active male subjects. In comparison to presupplementation values, a nonsignificant 2.4% increase in peak and mean power output was observed in the seventh 10 sec sprint following supplementation.

Burke et al. (1996) assigned 32 elite male and female swimmers from the Australian National Team to either a placebo or creatine monohydrate supplementation group (20 g/day for 5 days, 100 g total), evaluating their performance in a 2 × 10 sec sprint protocol before and after the supplementation period. The 2.3% increase in power and work observed following supplementation was not significant.

Cooke et al. (1995) assigned 12 untrained males to either a placebo or acute supplementation (20 g/day for 5 days, 100 g total) group in order to study the effects of creatine on maximal cycle sprint performance (2 × 15 sec tests). The bouts were separated by a 2 min recovery period. The authors reported no significant effect on peak power, time to peak power, total work, and an index of fatigue.

In a later study, Cooke and Barnes (1997) examined the effect of recovery interval on two maximal sprint bouts. Eighty healthy, active males were randomly assigned to either a placebo or acute supplementation (20 g/day for 5 days, 100 g total) group. Within each group, subjects were also randomly assigned to one of four recovery intervals (30, 60, 90, or 120 sec). The investigators reported that creatine supplementation demonstrated no apparent effect on power output during the second sprint bout for any of the recovery conditions.

Gonzalez de Suso et al. (1995) used a crossover design to investigate the effect of creatine supplementation (21 g/day for 14 days, 294 g total) on cycle sprint performance (7 bouts × 7 sec) in 19 trained males and females. Creatine supplementation increased muscle [PCr]/[ß-ATP] ratio as determined by ^{31}P-MRS. However, performance findings were equivocal, with a 7% increase in peak power output observed in the group that consumed the placebo followed by creatine, but no change in the group that consumed the creatine followed by the placebo. The length of the washout period was not clearly indicated and may have been too short. If so, a meaningful treatment effect might have been masked if there was a residual effect in the group that consumed creatine in the first trial.

Using a crossover design, Ledford and Branch (1999) investigated the effects of acute creatine supplementation (20 g/day for 5 days, 100 g total) vs. placebo (Polycose) on repeated Wingate test performance (3 × 30 sec with 5 min rest between sets) in nine trained females. Supplementation and placebo treatments were separated by a 90-day washout period. When post-placebo and post-creatine performances for the third Wingate test were compared for all subjects, increases of 1.8% (total work) and 7.9% (peak power) were noted, but there were no significant treatment or treatment-by-test interaction effects.

Stone et al. (1999) randomly assigned 42 American collegiate football players to five weeks of supplementation with either a high creatine dose (0.22 g/kg body mass per day [~20 g/day], ~700 g total), a low creatine dose (0.09 g/kg body mass per day [~8 g/day] plus pyruvate (~280 g total), an anhydrous water-soluble powder placebo, or a silica placebo. Subjects completed a cycle ergometer protocol consisting of 15 × 5 sec sprints prior to and after supplementation. Neither dose of creatine improved cycle ergometer sprint performance.

Among studies using short-term, high-intensity, repetitive cycle ergometer protocols, with time frames ranging from 6 to 30 sec, 18 showed a mean of 16% improvement (median = 7%) in performance following creatine supplementation. Seven studies did not support the ergogenicity of creatine supplementation in repetitive cycle ergometer tasks.

Studies Reporting Ergogenic Effects on Single-Bout Cycle Ergometer Tasks No studies using methods consisting of a single cycle ergometer bout protocol show improved performance following creatine supplementation. However, in their previously described study, Balsom et al. (1995) reported a 5% increase in power during a 10 sec sprint task after creatine supplementation (20 g/day for 5 days, 100 g total). It is important to note, however, that this single bout followed repeated bouts of fixed-intensity cycle ergometer exercise (5 × 6 sec with 30 sec recovery periods). Dawson et al. (1995) measured sprint performance (6 bouts $\times$ 6 sec with a 24 sec recovery period between bouts) in 22 subjects who were randomly assigned to either a placebo or acute supplementation (20 g/day for 5 days, 100 g total) group. In addition to the previously described increases in peak power output and total work after supplementation, the creatine group completed more work in sprint 1 (in isolation) than the placebo group, a finding also replicated by Kreider et al. (1998), suggestive that creatine supplementation may improve single-bout cycle ergometer performance.

Studies Reporting No Ergogenic Effects on Single-Bout Cycle Ergometer Tasks   Five studies show no ergogenic effect of creatine supplementation on single-bout cycle ergometer performance. Chetlin et al. (1998) compared the effects of two different creatine supplements on Wingate test performance using resistance settings of 10% and 12.5% of body mass. Thirty-three resistance-trained males were randomly assigned to one of three groups: 20 g creatine monohydrate per day for 10 days (200 g total), 10 g creatine monohydrate per day plus dextrose and adenosine for 10 days (100 g creatine total), or placebo. Neither level of creatine supplementation had an effect on Wingate test performance at either resistance.

Dawson et al. (1995) assigned 18 healthy, active males to either a placebo or short-term supplementation (20 g/day for 5 days, 100 g total) group to investigate the effects of creatine on a single sprint performance (10 sec). The 4.8% improvement in performance was not significant.

Odland et al. (1997) investigated the effect of creatine supplementation on Wingate test performance. Nine physically active males were studied in a single-group repeated-measures design. Wingate test power and work following creatine supplementation (20 g/day for 3 days, 60 g total) were compared to results for placebo and control treatments in a counterbalanced manner. An increase in muscle creatine uptake as measured by needle biopsy technique was observed. Using watts per kilogram as the measure of power, these investigators reported no significant differences between the trials in peak power, mean 10 sec power, or mean 30 sec power. Moreover, although biopsies of the vastus lateralis revealed a significantly higher [TCr]/[ATP] ratio in the muscle after creatine supplementation compared to placebo or control conditions, there was no difference in the [PCr]/[ATP] ratio, which may have been the basis for the insignificant findings in performance.

In another single-group repeated-measures design, Ruden et al. (1996) investigated the effect of creatine supplementation (20 g/day for 4 days) vs. placebo on Wingate test performance (1 $\times$ 30 sec) in nine college-aged subjects (five females, four males). Treatment order was counterbalanced, with only a 14-day washout between treatments. Peak power, mean power, and total work were unaffected by creatine supplementation. As previously discussed, a short washout period could have masked an ergogenic effect of creatine supplementation (Vandenberghe et al. 1997a; Ziegenfuss et al. 1998a).

Using a crossover design, Snow et al. (1998) examined the effect of acute supplementation (30 g/day for 5 days, 150 g total) on performance in a 20 sec single cycle sprint. Muscle [TCr] increased by 9.5% (11.8 mmol/kg dry mass), a small change compared with the increases reported by other investigators (Greenhaff et al. 1993a, 1994a, 1996, 1997b). There was no change in [PCr]. Compared to the placebo treatment, creatine supplementation did not improve sprint performance. The authors speculated that the smaller-than-expected increases observed were attributable to subjects who were "nonresponders" to creatine supplementation.

In general, studies have shown no significant effect of creatine supplementation on performance in single, maximal cycle ergometer exercise bouts of less than 30 sec, although some research has shown improvement in a single bout following a series of repetitive cycle bouts and even in the first bout of repetitive bouts.

Field Studies

The ultimate application of an ergogenic effect following creatine supplementation is improved performance of high-intensity, short-duration single or repetitive tasks in the field setting (i.e., the sports arena), or in a laboratory environment designed to mimic field conditions. It is important that research findings corroborate the efficacy of creatine supplementation in field tasks that are dependent on muscle [PCr]. To date, few data support the ergogenicity of creatine supplementation for high-intensity, short-duration performance tasks outside of the laboratory with the possible exception of isotonic resistance tests such as the 1-RM bench press, a laboratory test that may resemble competitive weightlifting. Studies of high-intensity, short-duration jumping, running, swimming, skating, and throwing performance following creatine supplementation are presented in tables 5.5 through 5.8.

Jumping Performance

Field studies of jumping performance following creatine supplementation are presented in table 5.5.

Studies Reporting Ergogenic Effects   Several studies have shown significant improvement in jumping performance following creatine supplementation. In a study of sprinters and jumpers using a continuous 45 sec jumping test, Bosco et al. (1997) randomly assigned 14 athletes to either a placebo or creatine-supplementation (20 g/day for 5 days, 100 g total) group. In this study, a 7% increase in work was observed in the first 15 sec of the test and a 12% increase during the second 15 sec period. No effect was observed in the third 15 sec period.

Goldberg and Bechtel (1997) investigated the effects of supplementation on vertical jump performance in varsity football and track athletes. Thirty-four athletes

Table 5.5 Effect of Creatine Supplementation on High-Intensity, Short-Duration (≤ 30 sec) Single or Repetitive Jumping Tasks Involving the Adenosine Triphosphate-Phosphocreatine (ATP-PCr) Energy System. Studies Are Arranged According to Ergogenic Effects.

Investigator	Year	Population	N	Gender	Design	Initial CM dose g × d = dose			Mode	Ergogenic effect?	%Δ	Comments
Bosco et al.	1997	Sprinters and jumpers	14	M	RDBPC	20	5	100	45 sec continuous jump test	Y	12	Increased work capacity during first 15 sec of the test (7%) with 12% increase from 15 to 30 sec.
Goldberg and Bechtel	1997	Varsity football and track athletes	34	M	RDBPC	3	14	42	Vertical jump	Y	2.6	% Δ in body mass index was used as a statistical covariate.
Stone et al.	1999	Football players	42	M	RDBPC	20	35	700	Static vertical jump force	Y	3.5	Comparison of creatine with creatine + pyruvate, anhydrous powder, and silica placebo.
Stout et al.	1999	Football players	24	M	RDBPC	21	5	105	Vertical jump	Y	N/A	Increased vertical jump after Phosphagen HP™ supplementation (5.6 cm) compared to placebo (1.3 cm).

(continued)

113

Table 5.5 *(continued)*

Investigator	Year	Population	N	Gender	Design	Initial CM dose g × d = dose			Mode	Ergogenic effect? %Δ	Comments
Kirksey et al.	1997	Track and field athletes	36	M/F	RDBPC	20	42	840	Vertical jump	N	
Miszko et al.	1998	NCAA IA softball players	14	F	RDBPC	25	6	150	Vertical jump	N	
Noonan et al.	1998b	College athletes	39	M	RDBPC	20	5	100	Vertical jump	N	
Stone et al.	1999	Football players	42	M	RDBPC	8	35	280	Static vertical jump force	N	
Stout et al.	1999	Football players	24	M	RDBPC	21	5	105	Vertical jump	N	

RDBPC = Randomized, double-blind, placebo control

were assigned to either a placebo or low-dose (3 g/day for 14 days, 42 g total) supplementation group. After supplementation, vertical jump performance, examined by ANCOVA with percentage change in body mass index as the covariate, was improved by 2.6%.

Studies Reporting Mixed Effects of Different Forms of Creatine on Jumping Performance   Stone et al. (1999) also examined vertical jump performance in their study of American football players. Forty-two athletes were assigned to 35 days of one of four supplements: high-dose creatine (0.22 g/kg body mass per day [~20 g/day], ~700 g total), low-dose creatine (0.09 g/kg body mass per day [~8 g/day], ~280 g total plus pyruvate,), an anhydrous water-soluble powder placebo, or silica placebo. The authors measured countermovement and static vertical jump performance prior to and following the 5-week regimen. Calculated static vertical jump power was greater following the high-dose treatment (3.5%) and anhydrous powder placebo (3.0%) compared to the low-dose creatine or silica placebo.

In another study of discordant results in football players, Stout et al. (1999) compared the effects of a supplement containing creatine monohydrate and glucose with a supplement containing creatine monohydrate, sodium and potassium phosphates, and taurine (Phosphagen HP™) on vertical jump performance in football players. Twenty-four athletes were randomly assigned to either creatine-glucose, Phosphagen HP™, or placebo control for 8 weeks of supplementation, during which they also were engaged in speed drills and resistive training. The authors stated that following Phosphagen HP™ supplementation, increase in vertical jump performance (5.6 cm) was significantly greater than placebo (1.3 cm). Compared to the placebo group, creatine monohydrate + glucose supplementation regimen (21 g/day for 5 days, then 10.5 g/day for 51 days) did not significantly increase vertical jump performance (5.1 cm), due in part to large intra-group variance. It was unclear if the increase in vertical jump performance following Phosphagen HP™ supplementation was significantly greater than the gain following creatine monohydrate + glucose supplementation. This study is somewhat difficult to interpret due to the discordant results observed between the two creatine-containing supplements.

Studies Reporting No Ergogenic Effects   Not all jumping studies, however, have reported improvements following creatine supplementation. Kirksey et al. (1997) studied the effects of a longer supplementation regimen (42 days) on power output. Thirty-six male and female collegiate track and field athletes were randomly assigned to either a placebo or creatine (0.3 g/kg per day [~20 g/day], 840 g total) group. Static and countermovement vertical jump (CMVJ) performance was measured using a force plate before and after the 6-week supplementation period. There was no apparent effect of creatine supplementation on vertical jump performance.

Miszko et al. (1998) randomly assigned 14 female NCAA Division IA softball players to a either placebo or supplementation (25 g/day for 6 days, 150 g total) group in order to examine the effects of short-term creatine loading on vertical jump and reach performance. Following supplementation, a 3% decrease in vertical displacement (42.7 cm pre- vs. 41.1 cm post) was observed in the creatine group.

A 4.7% decrease was also observed in the placebo group (48.3 cm pre- vs. 46 cm post) The authors reported that body mass increased significantly in both groups [creatine, 1 kg (1.4%); placebo, 0.8 kg (1.2%)] which may have contributed to the observed decrement in performance. Although the authors stated that no between or within-group differences were observed at any time in the study, examination of their results revealed baseline body mass to be 5.9 kg lower (65.5 vs. 71.4 kg), sum of three skinfolds to be 12.2 mm less (59.5 vs. 71.7 mm) and vertical jump height 5.6 cm higher (48.3 vs. 42.7 cm) in the placebo group compared to the creatine group. However, as there were no significant differences between the groups, the interpretation was that creatine supplementation neither improved nor impaired jumping performance.

Noonan et al. (1998b) studied the effects of short-term supplementation (20 g/day for 5 days, 100 g total) followed by 8 weeks of maintenance supplementation at either 100 mg/kg fat-free mass (~8.5 g/day, ~480 g total) or 300 mg/kg fat-free mass (~25.5 g/day, ~1420 g total) on vertical jump height in 39 male college athletes. Supplementation resulted in insignificant increases of 2 cm and 1 cm in vertical jump height of the 100 and 300 mg/kg groups, respectively.

Summary   The subjects in each of these studies were athletes participating in sports in which jumping ability and a high percentage of type IIb muscle fibers are determinants of success. It has been noted by Casey et al. (1996) that creatine is likely to be preferentially assimilated by type IIb fibers and that any ergogenic effect of creatine would be related to increased [PCr] in these fibers. From these studies, it would appear that creatine supplementation may enhance jumping performance in some, but not all, elite athletes participating in high-power sports. The efficacy of creatine supplementation in improving jumping performance remains uncertain. This equivocality is best illustrated by ergogenic and null results, respectively, for track and field athletes (Bosco et al. 1997; Kirksey et al. 1997) and football players (Goldberg and Bechtel 1997; Stout et al. 1999; Stone et al. 1999). It is possible, as suggested in the study by Miszko et al. (1998), that gains in body mass may be counterproductive and actually impair vertical jumping ability.

Five studies have shown significant improvement (mean = 8%; median = 7%) in jumping performance (vertical jump or repetitive jumping protocols) following creatine supplementation. However, three studies have reported no improvement, and two studies report both ergogenic and nonsignificant results. An excessive gain in body mass could possibly impair jumping performance.

Sprint Running Performance

The importance of muscle [PCr] in sprint performance is illustrated in a cross-sectional study by Hirvonen et al. (1987), who divided seven male sprinters into two groups with maximal sprint velocities of 10.07 and 9.75 m/sec, respectively. Groups were compared at 40, 60, 80, and 100 m maximal sprint velocity. The faster group had a higher rate of high-energy phosphate breakdown for 40, 60, and 80 m. Change in pH and [lactate] was not great enough to explain the decrease in speed over 100 m. Although creatine supplementation was not a part of the design, the observations from this study support the premise that sprint speed might be enhanced if muscle [PCr] is increased via creatine supplementation. Highlights of the field studies are presented in table 5.6.

Studies Reporting Ergogenic Effects   Five studies show improvement in sprint running performance following creatine supplementation. Aaserud et al. (1998) studied repetitive sprint performance in male handball players. Subjects were randomly assigned to either placebo or creatine supplementation (15 g/day for 5 days, 75 g total). Prior to and following the initial supplementation, subjects completed an 8 x 40-m maximal sprint test. For an additional 9 days, subjects then ingested 2 g/day of either creatine (18 g total) or placebo, after which they completed the sprint test for a third time. Following the initial supplementation, times were significantly reduced in the last three sprints for the creatine group compared to the corresponding sprints at baseline. The authors also reported that although the group by test interaction was not significant (p = 0.14), times in the last three sprints remained significantly faster following an additional 9 days of creatine supplementation compared to baseline. As an index of fatigue, the increase in time between the first and last sprint was significantly less in the creatine group following the initial (0.7 s) and additional supplementation (0.67 s) compared to baseline (0.9 s). No improvement was observed in the placebo group. The authors concluded that creatine supplementation improves repetitive sprint performance in well-trained handball players and that additional research is needed to determine if low-dose supplementation following an initial loading regimen can maintain improved performance.

Goldberg and Bechtel (1997) investigated the effects of supplementation on 40 yard (36.6 m) sprint performance in varsity football and track athletes. Thirty-four athletes were assigned to either a placebo or low-dose supplementation (3 g/day for 14 days, 42 g total) group. Subjects were tested at baseline, days 7, and 14 of supplementation. Although the authors report that a significant improvement in sprint performance was observed in the creatine group from baseline to day 14, they concluded that anaerobic performance was enhanced only in vertical jump performance, which was previously discussed.

Lefavi et al. (1998) investigated the effects of high-dose short-term supplementation (19 g/day for 5 days, 95 g total) followed by chronic low-dose supplementation (2.4 g/day for 42 days, 101 g total) on repeat 60 yd sprint speed in 11 position (i.e., non-pitcher) baseball players. After supplementation, increased sprint performance was observed in these athletes. It is unclear when during supplementation these increases were observed. The authors concluded that baseball players represent a population that might benefit from creatine supplementation.

In their comparison of two different maintenance doses (100 [~8.5 g/day] vs. 300 [~25.5 g/day] mg/kg fat-free mass for 8 weeks) following initial creatine loading (20

Table 5.6 Effect of Creatine Supplementation on High-Intensity, Short-Duration (≤ 30 sec) Single or Repetitive Running Performance Tasks Involving the Adenosine Triphosphate-Phosphocreatine (ATP-PCr) Energy System. Studies Are Arranged According to Ergogenic Results.

Investigator	Year	Population	N	Gender	Design	Initial CM dose g × d = dose			Mode	Ergogenic effect?	%Δ	Comments
Aaserud et al.	1998	Handball players	14	M	RDBPC	15 2	5 9	75 18	8 × 40 m maximal sprints	Y	N/A	Time faster in the last 3 sprints.
Goldberg and Bechtel	1997	Football and track athletes	34	M	RDBPC	3	14	42	40 yd (36.6 m)	Y		
Lefavi et al.	1998	Baseball players	11	M	RDBPC	19	5	95	Repeat 60 yd sprints	Y	N/A	Improved speed in non-pitcher position players.
Noonan et al.	1998b	College athletes	39	M	RDBPC	20	5	100	40 yd (36.6 m)	Y	1.13	Comparison of 100 mg/kg (8.5 g/d) and 300 mg/kg (25.5 g/d) doses. 100 mg group improved (5.3 to 5.24 sec) with no change in 300 mg group (5.23 to 5.19 sec).
Stout et al.	1999	Football players	24	M	RDBPC	21	5	105	100 yd (91.4 m) time	Y	N/A	Decrease in 100 yd time after Phosphagen HP™ (−0.31 sec)

compared to placebo (−0.02 sec).

Javierre et al.	1997	Sprinters	12	M	RDBPC	25	3	75	150 m time	N
Lefavi et al.	1998	Basketball players	37	M	RDBPC	19	5	95	Repeat 94 ft sprints	N
Miszko et al.	1998	NCAA IA softball players	14	F	RDBPC	25	6	150	30 yd (27.43 m) × 5 with 1 min rest	N
Redondo et al.	1996	Highly trained athletes	22	M/F	RDBPC	25	7	175	60 m sprint	N
Smart et al.	1998	National soccer players	11	M	RDBPC	24	6	144	30 × 20 m with 30 sec rest	N
Stout et al.	1999	Football players	24	M	RDBPC	21	5	105	100 yd (91.4 m) time	N
Thorensen et al.	1998	Soccer players	18	M	RDBPC	20	6	120	40 yd (36.6 m) × 6	N

RDBPC = Randomized, double-blind, placebo control

g/day for 5 days, 100 g total) in 39 male college athletes, Noonan et al. (1998b) reported a significant 1.1% improvement in 40 yd sprint time in the 100 mg/kg group (5.30 to 5.24 sec). Sprint performance in the 300 mg/kg group was also faster (5.23 to 5.19 sec), but the improvement was not statistically significant. It is important to note that the presupplementation time of the 300 mg/kg group (5.23 sec) was faster than the postsupplementation time of the 100 mg/kg group (5.24 sec), suggesting that the two groups might have had different sprint abilities.

Studies Reporting Mixed Effects of Different Forms of Creatine on Sprint Running Performance   In their study of college football players, Stout et al. (1999) also compared the effects of supplementation with creatine and glucose (21 g creatine monohydrate per day for 5 days, followed by 10.5 g/day for 51 days), Phosphagen HP™, and placebo on 100 yd dash (91.4 m) performance. Subjects were also engaged in resistive training and speed drills (four sessions per week). Following Phosphagen HP™ supplementation, 100 yd dash time decreased significantly (–0.31 sec) compared to that with placebo (–0.02 sec). In contrast, improvement in sprint time following creatine plus glucose (–0.24 sec) was not significantly different from placebo (–0.02 sec). It was unclear whether the improvement in sprint time following Phosphagen HP™ supplementation was significantly greater (–0.31 sec) than that observed after supplementation with creatine plus glucose (–0.24 sec).

Studies Reporting No Ergogenic Effects   In addition to the above study by Stout et al. (1999), the following six studies show no improvement in sprint running performance following creatine supplementation. Javierre et al. (1997) studied the effects of creatine supplementation (25 g/day for 3 days, 75 g total) on 150 m sprint time in sprinters. Creatine supplementation failed to improve 150 m sprint time. In addition to sprint performance in baseball players, Lefavi et al. (1998) studied the effects of creatine-supplementation on sprint performance in 16 college basketball players. High-dose short-term supplementation (19 g/day for 5 days, 95 g total) followed by chronic low-dose supplementation (2.4 g/day for 42 days, 101 g total) failed to improve 94 ft (28.7 m) sprint drill performance. The authors concluded that creatine supplementation has no apparent effect on speed in basketball players.

Miszko et al. (1998) randomly assigned 14 female college softball players to either a placebo or acute supplementation (25 g/day for 6 days, 150 g total). Sprint performance (5 sets × 27.4 m [30 yd]) was measured before and after supplementation. There was no improvement in sprint performance.

Redondo et al. (1996) matched 24 highly trained male soccer and female field hockey athletes actively involved in training and randomly assigned them, in pairs based on gender and sprint speed, to either a treatment or placebo group. The treatment involved the effect of creatine monohydrate supplementation (25 g/day for 7 days, 175 g total) on sprint velocity during various zones (20-30 m, 40-50 m, 50-60 m) of three successive 60 m dash trials, each trial interspersed with a 2 min recovery period. Subjects were videotaped with three high-speed cameras, and velocities were determined from the videotape. Two sessions were conducted, one before and one following the treatment protocol. A four-factor MANOVA (group, session, trial, zone) revealed no main or interaction effects for the groups, indicating that the creatine supplement did not enhance sprint performance with this particular protocol.

In a study of national-class soccer players, Smart et al. (1998) measured sprint performance (30 × 20 m with 30 sec rest interval) in 11 athletes before and after they received either placebo or acute creatine supplementation (24 g/day for 6 days, 144 g total). Following supplementation, there was no change in sprint performance. The authors speculated that the observed increase in body mass after supplementation may have affected sprint performance.

Thorensen et al. (1998) investigated the effects of creatine supplementation on repetitive 40 yd (36.6 m) sprint performance in intercollegiate soccer players. Eighteen athletes were randomly assigned to either placebo or supplementation (20 g/day for 6 days, 120 g total). Prior to and after supplementation, subjects were timed in 6 × 40 yd sprints. No improvement in sprint performance was observed after supplementation. The authors concluded that creatine supplementation has no effect on repeated 40 yd sprint performance.

Of 10 studies on the effect of creatine supplementation on sprint run performance, that is, single or repetitive bouts over distances ranging from 20 m to 150 m, five have shown improved performance while seven have not. Two of the 10 studies (Lefavi et al. 1998; Stout et al. 1997) reported both ergogenic and nonergogenic effects. No studies have shown an ergolytic effect.

Summary According to the available literature, sprint running performance in highly trained athletes after creatine supplementation is either improved (Aaserud et al. 1998; Goldberg and Bechtel 1997; Lefavi et al. 1998; Noonan et al. 1998b; Stout et al. 1999) or unaffected (Javierre et al. 1997; Lefavi et al. 1998; Miszko et al. 1998; Redondo et al. 1996; Smart et al. 1998; Stout et al. 1999; Thorensen et al. 1998). In two of the studies reporting significant sprint improvement, the initial loading regimen was followed by a maintenance regimen of at least 6 weeks (Lefavi et al. 1998; Noonan et al. 1998b). However, one of these studies (Lefavi et al. 1998) showed contrasting results—improved speed in baseball players but no improvement in basketball players. One study (Stout et al. 1999) reported contrasting results with different forms of creatine. The ability of creatine supplementation to improve sprint running speed remains controversial. However, no study has shown a decrement in sprint speed following creatine supplementation. As suggested in chapter 8, if subjects gain body mass, maintenance of the same speed with a greater body mass could be important for some athletes, such as running backs in American football.

Swimming Performance

Field studies of swimming performance have used either swim ergometer protocols or timed swim sprints in a pool. Several studies have evaluated the effect of creatine supplementation on multiple swim performance tasks and have reported both ergogenic and nonsignificant effects (Leenders et al., 1999; Peyrebrune et al., 1998). Studies on the effects of creatine supplementation on swimming performance are presented in table 5.7.

Studies Reporting Ergogenic Effects   In one of the few studies to investigate the effect of gender on the effectiveness of creatine, Leenders et al. (1999) randomly assigned 32 male and female NCAA Division IA swimmers for 14 days to either a placebo or creatine-supplementation (20 g/day for 6 days; 10 g/day for 8 days) group. Swimming velocity was measured twice weekly in interval work (6 × 50 m with 3 min rest). The authors reported that males improved 50 m swim velocity from 1.63 to 1.67 m/sec (2.5%), with no improvement in females. They concluded that creatine-supplementation may improve velocity during interval work of ~30 sec duration in male swimmers, but not female swimmers.

Peyrebrune et al. (1998) studied the effects of acute creatine supplementation (9 g/day for 5 days, 45 g total) on swim sprint interval performance (8 × 45.72 m [50 yd]) in 14 elite male swimmers. Based on urinalysis, a 67% retention of creatine was calculated. An attenuation in the decline in swim interval work was observed for all sprints. Total time of swimmers following supplementation (200.2 sec) was significantly less than before supplementation (204.3 sec). Creatine supplementation had no effect on performance of a single 50 yard (45 m) sprint. The authors concluded that creatine supplementation may be effective for improving repetitive sprint swim performance in elite swimmers.

Studies Reporting No Ergogenic Effects   Grindstaff et al. (1997) studied the effect of creatine supplementation (21 g/day for 9 days, 189 g total) on swim bench sprint test performance (3 × 20 sec maximal effort interspersed with 60 sec rest) in 18 male and female junior competitive swimmers. Although creatine supplementation did not result in improved peak power and total work, there was a trend toward a significant group-by-test interaction ($p = 0.06$) using the change in work (i.e., work = postsupplementation work minus presupplementation work) as the dependent variable. The authors discussed evidence of a greater change in work in the first sprint for the creatine group compared to the placebo group. It is important to note, however, that there were large standard deviations around these mean changes in work, suggesting the presence of considerable interindividual response with regard to repeated trials, which may have been attributed to assessing males and females together.

Five other studies show no improvement in swim performance after supplementation. Leenders et al. (1999) examined the effects of 14 days of creatine supplementation (20 g/day for 6 days, 10 g/day for 8 days, 200 g total) vs. placebo on 25 m swim velocity in 32 male and female NCAA Division IA swimmers. Swimming velocity was measured twice weekly in interval work (10 × 25 m with a 60 sec rest interval). Supplementation had no effect on 25 m swimming velocity. The authors concluded that maximal swim velocity in meters per second for interval work lasting 10 to 15 sec was unaffected by creatine supplementation.

Table 5.7 Effect of Creatine Supplementation on High-Intensity, Short-Duration (≤ 30 sec) Single or Repetitive Swimming-Related Performance Tasks Involving the Adenosine Triphosphate-Phosphocreatine (ATP-PCr) Energy System. Studies Are Arranged According to Ergogenic Effects.

Investigator	Year	Population	N	Gender	Design	Initial CM dose g × d = dose			Mode	Ergogenic effect?	%Δ	Comments
Leenders et al.	1999	NCAA IA swimmers	32	M/F	RDBPC	20 10	6 8	120 80	Swim velocity 6 × 50 m	Y	2.5	Velocity improved from 1.63 to 1.67 m/sec in males, with no change in females.
Peyrebrune et al.	1998	Elite swimmers	14	M	RDBPC	9	5	45	8 × 45 m sprint intervals	Y	2	Total swim time following creatine supplementation was 4.1 sec faster than before supplementation.
Grindstaff et al.	1997	Junior competitive swimmers	18	M/F	RDBPC	21	9	189	3 × 20 sec max swim bench	N		
Burke et al.	1996	Elite swimmers	32	M/F	RDBPC	20	5	100	25 m/ 50 m	N		
Leenders et al.	1999	NCAA IA swimmers	32	M/F	RDBPC	20 10	6 8	120 80	10 × 25 yd with 1 min rest	N		

(continued)

Table 5.7 *(continued)*

Investigator	Year	Population	N	Gender	Design	Initial CM dose g × d = dose			Mode	Ergogenic effect? %Δ	Comments
Leenders et al.	1996	Elite swimmers	6	F	RDBPC	20 10	6 8	120 80	10 × 25 yd (22.8 m) sprints	N	
Mujika et al.	1996	Swimmers	20	M/F	RDBPCX	20	5	100	25 m	N	
Peyrebrune et al.	1998	Elite swimmers	14	M	RDBPC	9	5	45	1 × 50 yd (45 m) sprint time	N	

RDBPC = Randomized, double-blind, placebo control
RDBPCX = Randomized, double-blind, placebo control, crossover

Burke et al. (1996) randomly assigned 32 elite swimmers to either placebo or supplementation (20 g/day for 5 days, 100 g total). Swim time for 25 m was measured prior to and after supplementation. There was no improvement in 25 m swim time following supplementation.

Leenders et al. (1996) studied the effects of creatine supplementation on average swim velocity during 25 m interval work. For 2 weeks, six female university swimmers consumed a placebo, after which they were randomly assigned to either placebo or creatine supplementation (20 g/day for 6 days, 10 g/day for 8 days, 200 g total) for 2 additional weeks. Subjects completed the following interval session: 10×25 yd (22.8 m) with each 25 yd at a 1 min interval, 1 time/week. There was no significant effect of creatine supplementation on repetitive, short-interval swim performance.

Using a crossover design, Mujika et al. (1996) randomly assigned 20 male and female swimmers to both placebo and supplementation (20 g/day for 5 days, 100 g total) regimens in a counterbalanced treatment order. Creatine was found to have no significant effect on 25 or 50 m swim performance, with times approximately 1% slower after supplementation.

In addition to examining the effects of creatine on swim interval performance, Peyrebrune et al. (1998) studied the effects of acute creatine supplementation (9 g/day for 5 days, 45 g total) on time in a single 50 yd swim sprint in 14 elite swimmers. After supplementation, slower times were reported in both groups (creatine: pre- = 22.95 ± 0.51 sec, post- = 23.24 ± 0.70 sec [1.3%]; placebo: pre- = 23.36 ± 0.50 sec, post- = 23.45 ± 0.58 sec [0.4%]) with no significant differences between groups. The authors reported that these times were significantly slower than the personal best performances of the swimmers. They concluded that while creatine supplementation may improve interval swim performance, it appears to have no effect on time for a single swim sprint.

Of six studies addressing the effect of creatine supplementation on sprint swim performance, that is, single or repetitive bouts over distances ranging from 25 to 50 m, two have shown improved performance whereas the remainder have not. Two studies reported an impaired swim performance, possibly associated with an increased body mass and resultant increase in body drag (Mujika et al. 1996; Peyrebrune et al. 1998). Two studies (Leenders et al. 1999; Peyrebrune et al. 1998) report both ergogenic and nonergogenic results following creatine supplementation.

Summary   The available literature on creatine supplementation and sprint swim performance is scant, with two of only five studies supporting the use of creatine in enhancement of swim performance. Two studies (Leenders et al. 1999; Peyrebrune et al. 1998) report both ergogenic and negative effects on swim performance following creatine supplementation. Two studies showed increased swim time (i.e.,

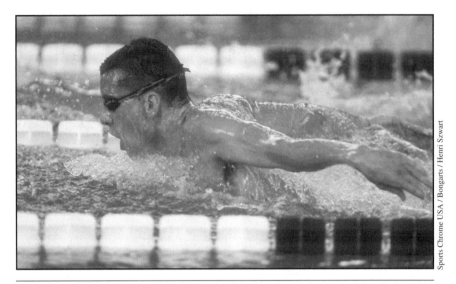

Sports Chrome USA / Bongarts / Henri Szwart

Figure 5.5   Swim sprints of 25-50 m represent one of the various field tests used to evaluate the ergogenic effects of creatine.

decreased performance) after creatine supplementation. Mujika et al. (1996) noted that impaired swim performance might be related to increased body mass, which could increase drag forces in swimming.

Miscellaneous Tasks

The effects of creatine supplementation on skating and throwing performance are presented in table 5.8.

Skating Performance   Two studies have provided contrasting results concerning the effects of creatine on speed skating performance time. Jones et al. (1998) assigned 16 elite ice hockey players to either a placebo or supplementation group. Supplementation consisted of an acute loading phase (20 g/day for 5 days, 100 g total) followed by a maintenance regimen (5 g/day for 10 weeks, 350 g total). Sprint performance (90 m skate sprint time every 30 sec with a 30 m split time) was measured prior to and after supplementation. Split time for 30 m was improved (3.6%) at both 10 days and 10 weeks of supplementation. Noonan et al. (1998a), however, reported that acute supplementation (20 g/day for 6 days, 120 g total) did not improve time to completion of a skating course.

The effects of creatine supplementation on ice skating performance are divergent: performance in 30 m sprint split times was improved, but time to complete a skating course was not improved.

Table 5.8 Effect of Creatine Supplementation on High-Intensity, Short-Duration (≤ 30 sec) Single or Repetitive Miscellaneous Skating or Throwing Performance Tasks Involving the Adenosine Triphosphate-Phosphocreatine (ATP-PCr) Energy System. Studies Are Arranged According to Ergogenic Effects.

Investigator	Year	Population	N	Gender	Design	Initial CM dose g × d = dose			Mode	Ergogenic effect?	%Δ	Comments
Goldberg and Bechtel	1997	Football and track athletes	34	M	RDBPC	3	14	42	Leg sled test	Y		
Jones et al.	1998	Elite ice hockey players	16	M	RDBPC	20 5	5 70	100 350	Timed 90 min skate sprint	Y	3.6	30 m split time was improved at 10 d and 10 wk following CM.
Noonan et al.	1998a	Ice hockey players	12	M	RDBPC	20	6	120	Timed skating course	N		
Lefavi et al.	1998	Baseball pitchers	10	M	RDBPC	19	5	95	Fastball pitching velocity × 5	N		

RDBPC = Randomized, double-blind, placebo control

Throwing   In addition to investigating sprint speed in position baseball and basketball players, Lefavi et al. (1998) studied the effects of creatine supplementation on the average speed of five fastballs in 10 baseball pitchers. Supplementation consisted of an initial loading phase of 19 g/day for 5 days (95 g total) with an additional 2.4 g/day for 42 days (101 g total). Creatine supplementation had no effect on velocity of fastball pitches in college baseball pitchers.

Creatine supplementation did not improve baseball pitching velocity.

Leg Sled Test   In their study of American football players and track athletes, Goldberg and Bechtel (1997) randomly assigned 34 subjects to either a placebo or supplementation group in order to study the effects of low-dose supplementation (3 g/day for 14 days, 42 g total) on lower body strength and power. During the study, subjects were concurrently engaged in off-season resistive training. Each subject completed a leg sled test using twice his body mass at baseline, 7 days, and 14 days of supplementation. Although the authors reported significant improvement in leg sled test performance in the creatine group at day 14 compared to baseline, they concluded that anaerobic performance was enhanced only in vertical jump performance which has been previously discussed in this chapter.

Performance Studies Including Biochemical Markers of Creatine Supplementation

Augmentation of the ATP-PCr energy system by creatine supplementation could help maintain cellular phosphagen energy charge, thereby reducing reliance on glycolysis, and decreasing production of lactate, ammonia (NH_3), and hypoxanthine during high intensity single-bout or repetitive high-intensity short duration tasks. Several of the previously discussed studies have measured various biochemical markers of energy metabolism such as blood [lactate], [NH_3] and [hypoxanthine] in addition to performance measures.

Isometric Strength and Endurance   In their study of congestive heart failure patients, Andrews et al. (1998) reported that creatine supplementation (20 g/day for 5 days, 100 g total) decreased post-exercise plasma [NH_3] and [lactate] in addition to improving isometric grip strength. The authors concluded that creatine supplementation attenuates the abnormal muscle responses seen in these patients.

The focus of a study of Greenhaff et al. (1993b) was the theory and mechanisms involved in phosphagen metabolism during an electrically evoked isometric stimulus. Twelve healthy males and females were assigned to placebo or acute-supplementation (20 g/day for 5 days, 100 g total) regimens, before and after which they underwent electrical stimulation designed to elicit isometric contractions of 1.6 sec duration with an equal rest interval. Following supplementation, muscle [PCr], measured following the contractions, was 20% higher as measured by needle biopsy technique and 11% higher with ^{31}P-MRS. The authors hypothesized that creatine may accelerate post-exercise PCr resynthesis. This possibility is certainly consistent with the observation, as documented throughout this chapter, that the ergogenicity of creatine seems to be more apparent in repetitive rather that single-bout exercise tasks.

Mihic et al. (1998) measured isometric maximal voluntary hand grip strength under ischemic conditions in order to study the possibility that creatine supplementation may increase plasma creatine kinase activity. Thirty healthy male and female subjects were randomly assigned to either placebo or creatine (20 g/day for 5 days, 100 g total) groups. Pre- and post-exercise blood samples were obtained before and after supplementation. Resting plasma [creatine kinase] and post-exercise [lactate] were unaffected by creatine supplementation.

Vandenberghe et al. (1999) reported that although creatine supplementation (5 g/day for 5 days) significantly increased resting muscle [PCr] after 2 and 5 days by 11% and 16% respectively, there was no significant effect of the supplementation protocol on PCr resynthesis during intermittent isometric muscle contractions. The isometric effort involved three contractions for each of the following time and percent of maximal voluntary contraction: 1 min (85% MVC); 1.5 min (75% MVC); and 2 min (65% MVC).

Isotonic Strength and Endurance   In their study of the effects of creatine (25 g/day for 7 days, 175 g total) on bench press and jump squat performance, Volek et al. (1997a) also measured blood [lactate], stress ([cortisol]) and steroid ([testosterone]) hormone response. Following supplementation, they reported a higher post-bench press [lactate] and a trend toward a lower post-squat [lactate]. [Testosterone] and [cortisol] were not significantly changed by creatine supplementation.

Isokinetic Strength and Endurance   In their study of the effect of creatine (20 g/day for 5 days, 100 g total) on isokinetic muscle torque, Greenhaff et al. (1993a) reported that the accumulation of plasma [NH$_3$] during exercise was decreased after creatine ingestion compared to the placebo. The authors concluded that the observed improvement in performance was due to accelerated skeletal muscle PCr resynthesis, resulting in greater PCr availability.

Cycle Erqometer Performance   Balsom et al. (1995) measured cycle ergometer power output and pedal frequency (5 × 6-sec bouts with 30 sec recovery followed by a single 10-sec bout) in seven subjects before and after creatine supplementation (20 g/day for 6 days, 120 g total). Following supplementation, the observed increased resistance to fatigue, measured by an attenuated decline in pedal frequency, was associated with increased [PCr] and decreased muscle [lactate].

Birch et al. (1994) reported that creatine supplementation (20 g/day for 5 days, 100 g total) did not affect [lactate], but did significantly lower plasma [NH$_3$] in response to high-intensity cycle ergometer (3 × 30 sec) exercise. The authors concluded that lower [NH_3] in response to increased power output and work suggests an enhanced state of ATP turnover in exercising muscle.

Dawson et al. (1995) also reported that although creatine supplementation (20 g/day for 5 days, 100 g total) increased peak power and total work during high-intensity cycle ergometer exercise (6 $\times$ 6 sec with 24 sec rest), blood [lactate] response was not significantly different from the placebo group. In addition, they reported no effect of creatine supplementation on blood [lactate] following a single sprint (10-sec) performance.

Earnest et al. (1998) reported that a single 10 g dose did not improve Wingate test performance (2 $\times$ 30 sec with 5 min rest) beyond that observed following the initial loading regimen (20 g/day for 5 days, 100 g total) or significantly affect the change in blood [lactate], [NH_3] or [hypoxanthine].

Kamber et al. (1999) compared the effects of creatine (20 g/day for 5 days, 100 g total) and placebo supplementation on blood [lactate] response to high-intensity cycle ergometer interval sprint performance (6 $\times$ 10 sec sprints with a 30 sec rest interval) in 10 well-trained sport students. Significantly lower blood [lactate] was observed following post-creatine supplementation sprints 5, 7, and 10. Furthermore, post-creatine supplementation blood [lactate] two minutes following completion of the sprint exercise (9.8 mmol/liter) was 9% lower than the 10.2 mmol/liter observed prior to supplementation.

Odland et al. (1997) administered three Wingate tests to nine males under three treatment conditions: control, post-placebo, and post-creatine supplemention (20 g/day for 3 days, 60 g total). Treatment order was counterbalanced among the subjects. There was no difference between the conditions in post-Wingate test blood [lactate] response.

Snow et al. (1998) examined the effect of short-term creatine supplementation (30 g/day for 5 days, 150 g total) on performance in a 20 sec single sprint. Following supplementation, there were no significant changes in blood [lactate], [NH_3] or [hypoxanthine].

Jumping Performance   In their study of jumping performance, Bosco et al. (1995) reported that creatine supplementation (5 g/day for 42 days; 210 g total) increased blood [lactate] in soccer players during the first 30 sec of a 45 sec jumping test.

Sprint Running Performance   At least three studies of sprint running performance discussed in this chapter included measurement of blood [lactate], [NH_3], [hypoxanthine]. Miszko et al. (1998) reported that blood [lactate] response to repetitive sprint performance (5 $\times$ 27.4 m [30 yd]) tended to decrease following creatine supplementation compared to baseline in female college softball players but the difference was not significant. Smart et al. (1998) reported no change in blood [lactate] or [hypoxanthine], measured after repetitive sprint performance (30 $\times$ 20 m with 30 sec rest interval) in 11 athletes who received either placebo or acute creatine supplementation (24 g/day for 6 days; 144 g total). Thorensen et al. (1998) reported no difference between a placebo group and a creatine-supplemented (20 g/

day for 6 days, 120 g total) group in blood [lactate] response following the sixth 40 yard (36.6 m) sprint in intercollegiate soccer players. There was no improvement in sprint performance in any of these studies.

Swimming Performance   Three studies of swim performance also measured blood [lactate] or [NH$_3$] following creatine supplementation. Burke et al. (1996) reported no difference in post-25 m swim blood [lactate] in elite swimmers receiving either a placebo or creatine supplementation (20 g/d for 5 days, 100 g total). Mujika et al. (1996) reported that creatine supplementation (20 g/d for 5 days, 100 g total) had no effect on post 25 m blood [lactate] or [NH$_3$] response in elite male and female swimmers. Peyrebrune et al. (1998) reported no effect of creatine supplementation (9 g/d for 5 days, 45 g total) on blood [lactate] or [NH$_3$] following either 8 $\times$ 50 yd (45.7 m) repetitive swim sprints or a single 50 yd sprint in elite swimmers.

Summary   Of the performance studies in this section which measured the effect of creatine supplementation on blood [lactate], the only reports of decreased [lactate] response are in congestive heart failure patients following isometric hand grip exercise (Andrews et al. 1998) and in physically active males following repetitive cycle ergometer exercise (Balsom et al. 1995; Kamber et al. 1999). Most of the other studies which measured lactate response to high-intensity exercise reported either no change or increased blood [lactate] (Bosco et al. 1995, Volek et al. 1997b) following creatine supplementation. Decreased plasma [NH$_3$] following supplementation has been reported in three studies (Andrews et al. 1998, Birch et al. 1994, Greenhaff et al. 1993a)

Chapter Summary

This chapter has detailed the results of 80 studies describing effects of creatine supplementation on performance of activities that rely primarily on the ATP-PCr energy system. Ergogenic effects of creatine were found in 50 of these studies, with nonergogenic effects reported in 42 of the studies. Numerous studies show both ergogenic and nonsignificant effects of creatine supplementation on performance (Dawson et al. 1995; Goldberg and Bechtel, 1997; Leenders et al. 1999; Kirksey et al. 1997; Lefavi et al. 1998, Noonan et al. 1998b; Peyrebrune et al. 1998; Stone et al. 1999; Stout et al. 1999; Vandenberghe et al. 1996a; 1997a; 1997b). Performance modes that appear to be more favorably affected after creatine supplementation include repetitive cycle ergometry (18 [75%] of 24 studies), isokinetic torque production (7 [50%] of 14 studies), and isotonic force production (17 [74%] of 23 studies). These significant results were almost exclusively obtained in a laboratory environment. An ergogenic effect of creatine (mean = 6%; median = 4%) was reported in 9 of the 19 field studies reviewed here. Evidence of increased power, torque, and strength following creatine ingestion is available from laboratory-based research. Although existing scientific data suggest creatine supplementation may be ergogenic for some types of sports performances, corroboration of the ergogenicity of creatine supplementation in a field setting remains elusive because of the many uncontrolled extraneous factors that affect actual athletic performance.

6

Ergogenic Effects of Creatine Supplementation on Anaerobic Endurance

Theoretically, increasing muscle [phosphocreatine, PCr] through creatine supplementation may enhance performance in high-intensity, anaerobic endurance exercise tasks of 30-150 sec duration through such mechanisms as buffering of acidity, mitigation of lactic acid formation, and reduction of reliance on anaerobic glycolysis as a replenishment source of adenosine triphosphate (ATP). There have been some investigations of the effect of creatine supplementation on such exercise tasks. This chapter reviews studies involving the effects of creatine monohydrate supplementation on laboratory-based cycle ergometer tasks as well as field-based tasks such as running, jumping, and swimming. Tables 6.1 to 6.5 present the key points from these studies, with more detail as available presented in the text. Unless otherwise indicated, the studies described in this chapter employed a double-blind placebo control design. The length of the washout period is provided in studies that employed a crossover design. As in the previous chapter, *within-group* percentage changes (supplemented group or condition prescore vs. postscore) in performance (either reported by the investigators or calculated from the available data as [(post-pre)÷pre-100]) are provided. Percentage change in a repetitive exercise protocol was calculated using the pre- and postsupplementation performances for the last bout. The method of measurement of muscle [creatine] (e.g., biopsy, ^{31}P-magnetic resonance spectroscopy [^{31}P-MRS], urinary creatine/creatinine excretion) is indicated for those studies which measured creatine uptake. Studies which included biochemical markers of energy metabolism in addition to performance variables (e.g., measurement of blood [lactate], ammonia ([NH_3]), [hypoxanthine]) will also be discussed.

> Theoretically, increasing muscle [PCr] through creatine supplementation may enhance performance in high-intensity, more prolonged exercise tasks of 30-150 sec duration through such mechanisms as buffering of acidity, mitigation of lactic acid formation, and reduction of reliance on anaerobic glycolysis as a replenishment source of ATP.

Studies involving the effect of creatine supplementation on high-intensity exercise tasks dependent primarily on anaerobic glycolysis—maximal tasks lasting approximately > 30 to ≤ 150 sec—are not as numerous as those involving the ATP-PCr energy system. However, some good data are available relative to related exercise tasks involving resistance exercise, cycle ergometer protocols, both laboratory and field running tests, and miscellaneous exercise tasks.

Resistance-Exercise Tasks

Four studies have addressed the effects of creatine supplementation on isometric, isotonic, and isokinetic resistance-exercise tasks lasting longer than 30 sec. These studies are presented in table 6.1.

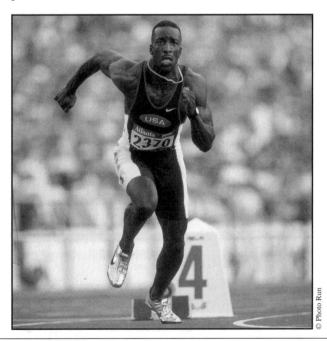

Figure 6.1 Some contend that creatine supplementation may reduce lactic acid production and help delay the onset of fatigue.

Table 6.1 Effect of Creatine Supplementation on High-Intensity, Prolonged-Duration (> 30 to ≤ 150 sec) Single or Repetitive Isometric (IM), Isotonic (IT), and Isokinetic (IK) Resistance-Exercise Tasks Involving the Anaerobic Glycolysis Energy System.

Investigator	Year	Population	N	Gender	Design	Initial CM dose g × d = dose			Mode/exercise	Ergogenic effect?	%Δ	Comments
Maganaris and Maughan	1998	Healthy	10	M	RDBPCX	10	5	50	IM	Time to exhaustion at 20%, 40%, 60%, 80% of MVC for knee extensors	Y	20 23 36 60	Improvement ranging from ~20% (20% of MVC) to ~60% (80% MVC).
Kurosawa et al.	1997	Healthy	5	M/F	SGRM	5	14	70	IM	Grip—30% MVC/sec to exhaustion	N		
Smith et al.	1998b	Young vs. middle aged	9	M	SGPC	20	5	100	IT	Leg exhaustion exercise (× 3); bouts 1-2, 2 min; bout 3 to exhaustion	Y	30	Resting and recovery [PCr] increased by 15% (young) and 30% (middle aged). Bout 3 time to exhaustion increased by 30%, 118 sec (pre-) vs. 154 sec (post-).
Ööpik et al.	1998	Karate	6	M	RDBPCX	20	5	100	IK	30 knee extensions (1.57 rad /sec, ~45 sec)	N		

RDBPCX = Randomized, double-blind, placebo control, crossover   SGPC = Single group, placebo control   SGRM = Single group, repeated measures

135

Isometric Exercise Tasks

The two studies of prolonged isometric force production after creatine supplementation present contrasting results. Maganaris and Maughan (1998) studied the effects of prolonged isometric contraction of the knee extensor muscles. Ten healthy males were randomly assigned to both placebo and creatine (10 g/day for 5 days, 50 g total) groups in a crossover design. Urinalysis revealed that ~35% of the ingested creatine was excreted during the supplementation period. As discussed in chapter 5, the authors noted an increase in maximal isometric knee extension force. However, they also reported an increase in isometric endurance, measured as time to fatigue in the dominant leg, at 80%, 60%, 40%, and 20% of maximal voluntary contraction (MVC). Examination of their data revealed the improvement to range from ~20% (20% of MVC) to ~60% (80% of MVC). Increased time to exhaustion was also observed at 80% of MVC in the nondominant leg for the group receiving placebo followed by creatine. The group receiving creatine first (days 2-6) retained significant increases in MVC for both the stronger and weaker legs following the placebo treatment (days 9-13). This residual effect was probably due to the short (3 day) washout between treatments. Significant improvements were observed only following creatine supplementation in the group which first received the placebo treatment. The authors concluded that muscle hypertrophy resulting from both resistance training and creatine supplementation may account for increased isometric endurance.

Using a single-group repeated-measures design, Kurosawa et al. (1997) investigated the effect of 2 weeks of isometric grip exercise resistance training of the nondominant arm combined with creatine supplementation (5 g/day for 14 days, 70 g total) on time to exhaustion at 30% of MVC at a rate of 1 contraction per second. Subjects were five healthy males and one female. Muscle creatine uptake was measured by ^{31}P-MRS. Nonsignificant improvements of 23% and 95% were reported for the nontrained, dominant arm (pre- = 81.3 sec; post- = 99.8 sec) and the trained, nondominant arm (pre- = 73.8 sec; post- = 144.3 sec; 95%), respectively. Although rather substantial, these changes presumably were not statistically significant because of the large variance and small sample size.

Isotonic Exercise Tasks

Smith et al. (1998b) compared the effects of creatine supplementation in young (< 40 years of age) and middle-aged (> 50 years of age) male and female subjects. In a single-blind manner, subjects ingested placebo followed by creatine (20 g/day for 5 days, 100 g total). Prior to each treatment, subjects performed an isotonic exercise protocol consisting of three leg extension sets. The first two sets were 2 min in duration at a rate of 37 contractions per second. The last set was performed at the same rate to exhaustion. Muscle [PCr] was measured by ^{31}P-MRS at rest and during the exercise. Creatine ingestion significantly increased resting and recovery [PCr] in both young (15%) and middle-aged (30%) subjects. For all subjects, time to exhaustion in the third set increased by 30% after creatine supplementation (118 sec to 154 sec). The authors concluded that creatine supplementation had a greater effect on [PCr] availability and resynthesis in middle-aged subjects. This is a unique and interesting finding in light of the fact that the population studied in the vast majority of the creatine-supplementation literature consists of young (≤30 years of age), physically active males.

Isokinetic Exercise Tasks

In an investigation of the potential for creatine supplementation to attenuate the loss of work capacity following loss of body mass, Ööpik et al. (1998) studied the effects of creatine supplementation (20 g/day for 5 days, 100 g total) on isokinetic force production in elite karate martial artists. Subjects, who had undergone rapid loss of body mass, received both placebo and creatine in a crossover manner. Isokinetic knee extension force production (30 knee extensions at 1.57 rad [90°]/sec^{-1} for 45 sec) was measured in subjects before and after creatine supplementation. Compared to placebo, creatine supplementation adversely affected the subjects' work capacity. The results of this study are relevant to sports such as wrestling and would indicate that reduced work capacity associated with rapid loss of body mass is not ameliorated by creatine supplementation. Confirming data are needed.

Summary of Resistance-Exercise Studies

The literature concerning the effect of creatine on high-intensity, longer duration resistance exercise is scant. Two of the four studies discussed in this section show improved performance in isometric (Manganaris and Maughan 1998) and isotonic (Smith et al. 1998b) exercise tasks of ≥ 30 sec duration. Another study of low-intensity isometric performance (Kurosawa et al. 1997) showed large percentages in improvement after supplementation that were not significant due to inadequate statistical power. Ööpik et al. (1998) reported an adverse effect of creatine on isokinetic performance following rapid loss of body mass—results that are intriguing but difficult to compare to those of the other studies. These studies support the conclusion that creatine supplementation may improve performance in high-intensity, longer duration resistive-exercise tasks.

Results are mixed regarding the effect of creatine supplementation on performance in isometric, isotonic, and isokinetic resistance-exercise tasks, with several studies showing an ergogenic effect and others no effect. Additionally, creatine supplementation did not prevent the decrease in isokinetic muscle performance normally observed in athletes undergoing significant body weight loss for competition.

Laboratory-Based Cycle Ergometer Studies

Studies of the effects of creatine on high-intensity, prolonged cycle ergometer performance are presented in table 6.2. Four studies show increased cycle ergometer performance (mean = 14%; median = 13%) following creatine supplementation. Jacobs et al. (1997) randomly assigned 26 male and female subjects to either a placebo or creatine monohydrate supplementation (20 g/day for 5 days, 100 g total) group. Subjects were tested on a cycle ergometer, riding to exhaustion at 125% of maximal oxygen consumption ($\dot{V}O_{2max}$). The investigators reported that ride time to exhaustion was increased significantly after creatine monohydrate supplementation from 131 to 143 sec (8.5%), while the time for the placebo group remained unchanged at 128 sec. Additionally, creatine monohydrate supplementation significantly increased by 9% the maximal accumulated oxygen deficit (difference between the oxygen demand of the work, (calculated from the $\dot{V}O_2$/power output relationship, and the cumulative $\dot{V}O_2$). The authors concluded that creatine supplementation may have an ergogenic effect on moderately prolonged anaerobic exercise tasks.

Prevost et al. (1997) randomly assigned 18 physically active college students to either placebo or creatine (18.75 g/day for 5 days [94 g total], then 2.25 g/day for 6 days [13.5 g total]). Before and after supplementation, subjects completed four different cycle ergometer protocols at 150% of $\dot{V}O_{2max}$, one of which was ≤150 sec in duration. After supplementation, time to exhaustion for continuous, nonstop riding increased by 24% (48 to 60 sec).

Nelson et al. (1998) examined the effect of creatine supplementation (20 g/day for 7-8 days, 140-160 g total) on anaerobic threshold during cycle ergometer graded exercise testing in 28 trained adults. The treatments were administered in an ordered manner, with the non supplemented condition preceding the creatine condition. Anaerobic threshold was defined as the rate of oxygen consumption ($\dot{V}O_2$) at the intersection of the high and low slope portions of the $\dot{V}_E/\dot{V}O_2$ relationship. Following creatine supplementation, the anaerobic threshold occurred at a significantly greater $\dot{V}O_2$ (2.5 1/min, 67% of peak $\dot{V}O_2$) compared to the nonsupplemented condition (2.2 1/min). The authors concluded that creatine supplementation altered the impact of different energy systems during exercise and, by shifting the anaerobic threshold, increased the subjects' ability to do purely aerobic work.

Smith et al. (1998a) randomly assigned 15 active but untrained males and females to either a placebo or acute supplementation (20 g/day for 5 days, 100 g total) group. Before and after supplementation, subjects completed two cycle ergometer exercise bouts to fatigue. After supplementation, an increase in time to exhaustion was observed at a work rate of 5.2 W/kg body mass (93 to 103 sec, 10.8%). The authors attributed these increases in anaerobic capacity to enhanced ATP resynthesis secondary to increased contribution from increased [PCr].

Three studies show no effect of creatine supplementation on cycle ergometer work of ≥ 60 sec. Using a single-group repeated-measures design, Febbraio et al. (1995) examined the effects of creatine supplementation (20 g/day for 5 days, 100

Table 6.2 Effect of Creatine Supplementation on High-Intensity, Prolonged-Duration (> 30 to < 150 sec) Single or Repetitive Cycle Ergometer Tasks Involving the Anaerobic Glycolysis Energy System.

Investigator	Year	Population	N	Gender	Design	Initial CM dose g	× d	= dose	Mode	Ergogenic effect?	%Δ	Comments
Jacobs et al.	1997	Physically active	26	M/F	RDBPC	20	5	100	125% VO_{2max}	Y	8.5	Maximal accumulated O_2 debt (MAOD) = predicted−actual VO_{2max}. 8.5% and 9% increases in time to exhaustion and MAOD.
Nelson et al.	1998	Trained athletes	28	M/F	SGRM	20	7-8	140-160	Anaerobic threshold	Y	13.6	Increase in anaerobic threshold from 2.2 L min to 2.5 L min.
Prevost et al.	1997	Physically active college students	18	M/F	RSBPC	18.75 2.25	5 6	94 13	Time to exhaustion at 150% VO_{2max}	Y	24	Increase in non stop time from 48 sec (pre-) to 60 sec (post-).
Smith et al.	1998a	Active untrained	15	M/F	RDBPC	20	5	100	Time to exhaustion at 5.2 W/kg	Y	10.8	Increase from 93 to 103 sec.
Febbraio et al.	1995	Untrained	6	M	SGRM	20	5	100	4 × 60 sec; 115-125%	N		

(continued)

Table 6.2 (continued)

Investigator	Year	Population	N	Gender	Design	Initial CM dose g × d = dose			Mode	Ergogenic effect? %Δ	Comments
Febbraio (cont.)									$\dot{V}O_{2max}$; 5th bout to exhaustion		
Schneider et al.	1997	Untrained	9	M	SBPC	7	25	175	5 × 60 sec	N	
Vanakoski et al.	1998	Trained athletes	7	M/F	SGRM	300 mg/kg/day	3	N/A	Maximal pedal speed; total work	N	

RDBPC = Randomized, double-blind, placebo control
RSBPC = Randomized, single-blind, placebo, control
SGPC = Single group, placebo control
SGRM = Single group, repeated measures

g total) on cycle ergometer performance (4 × 60 sec sprints followed by a fifth bout to exhaustion, all at 115-125% of $\dot{V}O_{2max}$) in six active but untrained male subjects. Subjects were retested after a 28-day washout; during the last 5 days of this period, a placebo was consumed. An increase in intramuscular [total creatine, TCr] was observed following creatine supplementation, but there were no differences in duration of the fifth exercise bout between baseline, postsupplementation, and postwashout trials. Although the supplementation dose was sufficient to increase muscle [TCr], 28 days without supplementation was considered to be a sufficient time for muscle [TCr] to return to baseline. Compared to the value for the third presupplementation familiarization trial, creatine ingestion resulted in a 16% decrease in time to exhaustion. Thus, it would appear that subjects fatigued more quickly following creatine supplementation. The investigators concluded that creatine supplementation has no ergogenic effect on exercise performance when the ATP-PCr energy system is not the principal energy source.

Of seven studies involving the effects of creatine supplementation on high-intensity, prolonged cycle ergometer performance (30-150 sec), four showed increased cycle ergometer performance (mean = 14%; median = 13%), whereas three reported no significant effect.

Schneider et al. (1997) also studied the effects of creatine supplementation on nine untrained males, using a single-group, sequential treatment order design. Subjects ingested 25 g of creatine monohydrate per day for 7 days (175 g total). Before and after supplementation, subjects completed cycle ergometer interval exercise consisting of 5 × 60 sec work intervals. Creatine exerted no beneficial effect on cycle ergometer work in these subjects.

Vanakoski et al. (1998) compared the effects of a single dose of caffeine (7 mg/kg body mass), creatine (300 mg/kg body mass/day for 3 days), caffeine plus creatine, and placebo on anaerobic exercise performance in seven trained athletes. Creatine uptake was confirmed by monitoring plasma [creatine] over time. Approximately 70 min after drug administration, subjects completed 3 × 1-min cycle ergometer exercise bouts at maximal speed. The authors reported no significant difference in heart rate response, maximal pedal rate (revolutions/min), maintenance of maximal speed, or total work (kJ) among the four treatments. The authors concluded that neither anaerobic performance nor post-exercise recovery was significantly affected by creatine supplementation.

Summary

To our knowledge, there are seven studies of the effects of creatine on high-intensity, more prolonged cycle ergometer performance. The four studies showing improved performance after creatine supplementation entailed groups described as

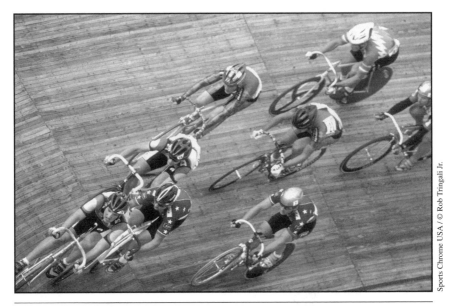

Sports Chrome USA / © Rob Tringali Jr.

Figure 6.2 If laboratory studies indicate that creatine supplementation may improve cycle ergometer performance, athletes such as pursuit cyclists might benefit.

"physically active" or "active, but untrained." Null findings were reported in the three studies that used "untrained" subjects. Only one study included a low maintenance dose (Prevost et al. 1997) in addition to the initial loading regimen. The literature is both scant and equivocal regarding the efficacy of creatine supplementation on cycle ergometer tasks that rely primarily on anaerobic glycolysis.

Running Performance

Studies of the effects of creatine supplementation on high-intensity, prolonged running performance under both laboratory and field conditions are presented in table 6.3.

Laboratory-Based Running Performance

Two studies of the effect of creatine on laboratory-based running tasks show increased performance following supplementation. As part of their study on jumping performance in sprinters and jumpers, Bosco et al. (1997) reported a 13% increase in treadmill running (20 km/hr at 5% incline) time to exhaustion (~60 sec) following creatine supplementation (25 g/day for 7 days, 175 g total).

Table 6.3 Effect of Creatine Supplementation on High-Intensity, Prolonged-Duration (> 30 to ≤ 150 sec) Single or Repetitive Running Tasks Involving the Anaerobic Glycolysis Energy System.

Investigator	Year	Population	N	Gender	Design	Initial CM dose g × d = dose			Mode	Ergogenic effect?	%Δ	Comments
Bosco et al.	1997	Sprinters/jumpers	14	M	RDBPC	20	5	100	Treadmill (20 km/hr at 5% grade) (~60 sec)	Y	13.2	Increase in time to exhaustion.
Earnest et al.	1997	Males	11	M	RDBPC	20	4	80	90 sec treadmill test (× 2)	Y	3.2	Increase in time to exhaustion for both 1st (1.5 sec) and 2nd (3.2 sec) runs.
Larson et al.	1998	Soccer players	14	F	RDBPC	15 5	7 84	105 420	Shuttle run (274.3 m)	Y	N/A	12 wk maintenance dose 5 g/d followed initial regimen. Shuttle run improved at 3-5 wk, with no further change.
Viru et al.	1994	Middle distance runners	10	M	RSBPC	30	6	180	4 × 300 m interval (90-95% max velocity)	Y	1	0.3 sec decrease in best 300 m interval time; improved total time.
Terrillion et al.	1997	Runners	12	M	RDBPC	20	5	100	700 m run	N		

RDBPC = Randomized, double-blind, placebo control   RSBPC = Randomized, single-blind, placebo control

143

Earnest et al. (1997) used a treadmill run test to exhaustion (approximately 90 sec) to investigate the effect of creatine monohydrate supplementation at 20 g/day for 4 days (80 g total), followed by 10 g/day for 6 days (60 g total), on intermediate-length anaerobic performance. Eleven male subjects assigned to either the supplement or placebo group trained specifically for the treadmill tests for two weeks; both pre- and postsupplementation trials were then administered. Subjects were tested twice during each trial, with each test being separated by an 8 min recovery period. An increase in total time to exhaustion (4.7 sec), as well as in time to exhaustion in the second exercise bout (3.2 sec), was observed following supplementation. The investigators concluded that creatine monohydrate supplementation may improve performance in longer anaerobic interval work.

Field-Based Running Performance

Three investigations of the effects of creatine on interval running performance outside of the laboratory have yielded contrasting results. Viru et al. (1994) tested 10 trained middle distance runners, equally assigned to either a placebo or creatine (30 g/day for 6 days, 180 g total) group, on separate days prior to and following supplementation. The test involved 4 × 300 m runs with a 4 min recovery between repetitions. The authors reported an enhanced performance in total time for the interval session, as well as a decrease in the final 300 m (0.3 sec, 1%), following creatine supplementation. They suggested that the increased use of PCr during exercise may contribute to the buffering of hydrogen ions.

Larson et al. (1998) provided 14 female soccer players with either placebo or a high-dose creatine-loading regimen (15 g/day for 7 days, 105 g total) followed by a low-dose maintenance regimen (5 g/day for another 12 weeks, 420 g total). Performance of a 274.3 m (300 yd) anaerobic shuttle run was improved 3 to 5 weeks after the initial loading regimen, but no further improvements were observed.

Terrillion et al. (1997) investigated the effects of creatine supplementation (20 g/day for 5 days, 100 g total) on interval running performance in male runners. Twelve subjects completed an interval workout (2 × 700 m) before and after receiving either creatine or a placebo. Creatine supplementation failed to improve 700 m run time in either of the two runs.

Summary of Running Studies

As is the case with cycle ergometer performance, there are relatively few studies on the effect of creatine supplementation on running tasks that rely primarily on anaerobic glycolysis. Four studies show improved performance (mean = 6%; median = 3%) following creatine supplementation, while one revealed no ergogenic effect. At this time, there appears to be some research support for improvement in high-intensity, more prolonged running performance following creatine supplementation.

Of five studies addressing the effect of creatine supplementation on prolonged, high-intensity laboratory or field running performance, four show improved performance (mean = 6%; median = 3%) whereas one shows no ergogenic effect.

Swimming Performance

Five studies of the effects of creatine supplementation on high-intensity, prolonged swimming performance are presented in table 6.4. One study reported mixed effects, whereas the remainder reported no significant ergogenic effect of creatine supplementation. Leenders et al. (1996) studied the effects of creatine supplementation on average swim velocity during 50 m and 100 m interval work. For 2 weeks, six female university swimmers consumed a placebo, after which they were randomly assigned to either placebo or creatine supplementation (20 g/day for 6 days; 10 g/day for 8 days) for 2 additional weeks. Subjects completed the following interval sessions: 6 $\times$ 50 m at a 3 min interval, 2 times/week; 12 $\times$ 100 m at a 2.5 min interval, 1 time/ week. The investigators reported a significant treatment (placebo vs. creatine) by time interaction, with an increase in average 50 m swim velocity from 1.54 to 1.6 m/ sec for the creatine group compared to no change in the placebo group. No treatment, time, or interaction effects were observed in average 100 m swim velocity. The authors concluded that 2 weeks of creatine supplementation may increase swim performance in interval training where the exercise interval is 30 to 35 sec.

Burke et al. (1996) examined the effect of creatine supplementation (20 g/day for 5 days, 100 g total) on 100 m swim time in 32 elite male and female swimmers who were assigned to either a placebo or creatine group. Creatine supplementation failed to improve 100 m sprint swim time. In a similar study, Mujika et al. (1996) assigned 20 male and female elite swimmers to either a placebo or creatine-supplementation (20 g/day for 5 days, 100 g total) group in a randomized double-blind manner. Creatine supplementation not only failed to improve swim time, but actually tended to impair performance in both the 50 m and 100 m.

In their study of male and female junior competitive swimmers, Grindstaff et al. (1997) randomly assigned subjects by matched pairs to either a placebo or creatine-supplementation (21 g/day for 9 days, 189 g total) group. Times for three heats of both 50 m and 100 m freestyle swim distance were measured before and after supplementation. Significant group (placebo, creatine)-by-time (pre-: Heats 1, 2, and 3; post-: Heats 1, 2, and 3) interactions were reported for both 50 m ($p = 0.04$) and 100 m ($p = 0.04$) swim time; these were largely explained by slower postsupplementation swim times in the placebo group. Although it was concluded that the study provided some evidence of the efficacy of creatine in enhancing repetitive swim sprint performance, supplementation had no effect on cumulative 50 m or 100 m swim time.

Peyrebrune et al. (1998) provided 14 elite swimmers with either placebo or low-dose creatine supplementation (9 g/day for 5 days, 45 g total). Creatine did not improve 45 m sprint time, which was reported to be 1.3% slower following supplementation. Finally, Thompson et al. (1996) randomly assigned 10 college-aged female competitive swimmers to either a placebo or creatine group in order to study the effects of a low-dose creatine supplementation regimen (2 g/day for 56 days) on 100 m swim performance. Using ^{31}P-MRS and near-infrared spectroscopy, the authors measured [PCr], [PCr]/[ß-ATP] ratio, and [ADP] at rest and during exercise (plantar flexion) both before and after supplementation. Creatine supplementation had no effect on muscle metabolites. Compared to the placebo, creatine supplementation was also ineffective in improving 100 m swim time.

Summary of Swimming Studies

Although more research is needed on the effect of creatine on high-intensity, longer-duration swimming performance, these studies indicate that supplementation is ineffective in improving swim time for distances of 50 to 100 m. Mujika et al. (1996) and Peyrebrune et al. (1998) report tendencies toward impaired performance following supplementation, an observation possibly related to increased drag secondary to increased body mass.

Of all studies addressing the effect of creatine supplementation on high-intensity, prolonged swimming performance, one reported a significant ergogenic effect, and five studies reported no ergogenic effect.

Miscellaneous Exercise Tasks

Table 6.5 presents three studies, one of prolonged jumping ability (Bosco et al. 1997), one of kayaking performance (McNaughton et al. 1998), and one of obstacle course performance (Ensign et al. 1998).

In contrast to findings for short-duration (≤30 sec) very high intensity activity, creatine supplementation is somewhat less likely to enhance performance of high-intensity, more prolonged (30 to 150 sec) tasks in either laboratory or field settings. Ergogenic effects have been documented for laboratory-based cycle ergometry and both laboratory and field running tests, but not for swimming performance. The lesser incidence of an ergogenic effect is probably explained by energy system specificity; that is, the ergogenic potential of creatine supplementation appears to be limited in tasks that rely primarily on anaerobic glycolysis for ATP synthesis.

Table 6.4 Effect of Creatine Supplementation on High-Intensity, Prolonged-Duration (> 30 to ≤ 150 sec) Single or Repetitive Swimming Tasks Involving the Anaerobic Glycolysis Energy System.

Investigator	Year	Population	N	Gender	Design	Initial CM dose $g \times d$ = dose			Mode	Ergogenic effect?	%Δ	Comments
Burke et al.	1996	Elite swimmers	32	M/F	RDBPC	20	5	100	100 m time	N		
Grindstaff et al.	1997	Junior competitive swimmers	18	M/F	RDBPC	21	9	189	3 × 100 m freestyle cumulative time; 3 × 50 m freestyle cumulative time	N		
Leenders et al.	1996	Elite swimmers	6	F	RDBPC	20 10	6 8	120 80	6 × 50 m at 3 min interval 12 × 100 m at 2.5 min interval	Y	3.9	Improvement in 50 m swim velocity from 1.54 to 1.6 m/ sec. No improvement in 100 m swim velocity.
Mujika et al.	1996	Swimmers	20	M/F	RDBPC	20	5	100	50 m time 100 m time	N		
Peyrebrune et al.	1998	Elite swimmers	14	M	RDBPC	9	5	45	45 m sprint	N		

(continued)

Table 6.4 *(continued)*

Investigator	Year	Population	N	Gender	Design	Initial CM dose g × d = dose			Mode	Ergogenic effect? %Δ	Comments
Thompson et al.	1996	Swimmers	10	F	RDBPC	2	42	84	100 m time	N	

Table 6.5 Effect of Creatine Supplementation on Miscellaneous High-Intensity, Prolonged-Duration (> 30 to ≤ 150 sec) Single or Repetitive Tasks Involving the Anaerobic Glycolysis Energy System.

Investigator	Year	Population	N	Gender	Design	Initial CM dose g × d = dose			Mode	Ergogenic effect? %Δ	Comments
Bosco et al.	1997	Sprinters/jumpers	14	M	RDBPC	20	5	100	45 sec maximal continuous jumping	N	
Ensign et al.	1998	U.S. Navy Seals	24	M	RDBPC	20	5	100	Field test (obstacle course)	N	
McNaughton et al.	1998	Elite kayakers	16	M	RDBPC	20	5	100	Kayaking; 90 sec work; 150 sec work	Y 16.2 13.6	3.3 kJ increase in work after supplementation. 3.9 kJ increase in work after supplementation.

RDBPC = Randomized, double-blind, placebo control

Jumping Performance

The study of Bosco et al. (1997), discussed in chapter 5, is included in this section as well because the duration of the jumping task exceeded 30 sec. The authors compared the effects of creatine supplementation (25 g/day for 7 days, 175 g total) and placebo on maximal continuous jumping ability in sprinters and jumpers. As noted previously, creatine supplementation resulted in performance improvements during 0 to 15 sec (7%) and 15 to 30 sec (12%) of the 45 sec maximal continuous jumping test. However, the authors do not report improvements in the final 15 sec of the test.

> Creatine supplementation has not been shown to improve high-intensity, prolonged (45 sec) jumping performance.

Kayaking Performance

McNaughton et al. (1998) randomly assigned 16 elite male kayakers to either a placebo or supplementation (20 g/day for 5 days, 100 g total) group in order to investigate the effects of creatine on work performance during 90 sec and 150 sec kayak ergometer tests. Compared to placebo, creatine supplementation resulted in increased work capacity for both the 90 sec test (3.3 kJ increase, 16.2%) and 150 sec test (3.9 kJ increase, 13.6%). The authors concluded that creatine supplementation can increase kayak ergometer anaerobic work output.

> Creatine supplementation has been shown to improve performance in kayaking performance tests of 90-150 sec.

Obstacle Course Performance

Ensign et al. (1998) randomly assigned 24 U. S. Navy Seals to either placebo or acute supplementation (20 g/day for 5 days) in order to investigate improvement in obstacle course performance. Although postsupplementation time to completion (115.4 sec) was 7% faster than presupplementation time (124.2 sec), this improvement was not statistically significant.

Performance Studies Including Biochemical Markers of Creatine Supplementation

Isokinetic Performance

Studying the effect of creatine supplementation on isokinetic performance during rapid body weight loss in six elite male karate athletes, Ööpik et al. (1998) also measured [lactate], [NH$_3$], [glucose], and [urea]. Subjects were assigned to either a placebo or creatine group (20 g/day for 5 days, 100 g total), during which they attempted to lose 5% of their body mass. Mass decreased significantly in both groups, with a greater loss in the placebo group (3.3 kg) compared to the creatine group (2.2 kg). Both groups experienced similar decreases in plasma volume (calculated from changes in hemoglobin and hematocrit). Following loss of body mass, post exercise [NH$_3$] and [lactate] were not significantly different between the groups.

Cycle Ergometer Performance

Nelson et al. (1998) measured blood [lactate] and [NH$_3$] in 28 trained males and females following graded exercise testing. Subjects completed a baseline exercise test in a nonsupplemented condition, with a second test following a supplementation period (20 g/day for 7-8 days, 140-160 g total). Blood samples were obtained prior to exercise, at 6 and 12 minutes of exercise, at test termination, and 5 minutes of post exercise recovery. They reported significantly lower exercise and recovery [lactate] and [NH$_3$] following supplementation compared to baseline.

Prevost et al. (1997) studied the effects of creatine supplementation (18.75 g/day for 5 days [94 g], then 2.25 g/day for 6 days, [13.5 g] ; 107.5 g total) on blood [lactate] following cycle ergometer time to exhaustion at 150% of $\dot{V}O_{2max}$. Following supplementation, immediate- and 3 minute post exercise blood [lactate] were significantly lower compared with presupplementation values. The authors concluded that decreased [lactate] following creatine supplementation may reflect decreased acidity, decreased reliance on anaerobic glycolysis, and increased resistance to fatigue. Febbraio et al. (1995) examined the effects of creatine supplementation (20 g/day for 5 days, 100 g total) on blood [lactate] and plasma [NH$_3$] before and following cycle ergometer exercise (4 × 60 sec bouts followed by a fifth bout to fatigue at 115-125% of $\dot{V}O_{2max}$). There were no differences in postexercise [lactate] and [NH$_3$] between creatine, familiarization, and control conditions.

Schneider et al. (1997) measured blood [lactate] response to repetitive cycling in nine untrained males (5 × 15 sec maximal bouts). Subjects received, in an ordered manner, placebo followed by creatine supplementation (25 g/day for 7 days, 175 g total), with treatments separated by 2 weeks. There was no difference between placebo and creatine treatments in blood [lactate] following each of the five cycle ergometer bouts.

Vanakoski et al. (1998) also measured blood [lactate] in their comparison of the effects of caffeine (a single 7 mg/kg dose), creatine (300 mg/kg body mass/day for 3 days), creatine plus caffeine, and placebo on anaerobic cycle ergometer performance (3 × 1 min bouts at maximal speed). There were no differences in blood [lactate] between the four treatments. In addition, caffeine pharmacokinetics were not affected by creatine ingestion.

Jumping and Running Performance

Bosco et al. (1997) measured the highest blood [lactate] observed following treadmill running to exhaustion (20 km/hr) and a 45 sec jumping test. Subjects were sprinters and jumpers who were assigned to either a placebo or supplementation (20 g/day for 5 days, 100 g total) group. Post-run [lactate] was significantly higher following supplementation compared to the baseline value. There was no significant change in post-jumping test [lactate] following supplementation compared to the baseline value.

In their study of treadmill running to exhaustion, Earnest et al. (1997) reported an increase in [lactate] following creatine supplementation in addition to increased time to exhaustion. The observation of increased [lactate] is inconsistent with the hypothesis that creatine supplementation may decrease reliance on anaerobic glycolysis and thereby attenuate an increase in [lactate].

Terrillion et al. (1997) measured blood [lactate] following interval running (2 × 700 m intervals with a 60 sec rest) in 12 competitive male runners who were assigned to either a placebo or creatine supplementation (20 g/day for 5 days, 100 g total) . There were no group, time (presupplementation vs. postsupplementation), or interval (bout 1 versus bout 2) effects on blood [lactate].

Swimming Performance

Burke et al. (1996) measured blood [lactate] following a 100 m sprint swim in 32 elite male and female swimmers who were assigned to either a placebo or creatine supplementation (20 g/day for 5 days, 10 g total). For both placebo and creatine groups, blood [lactate] was significantly lower following supplementation compared to baseline. There was no differences between the groups. The authors reported a trend toward a significant group-by-trial interaction ($p = 0.06$). The difference between presupplementation and postsupplementation [lactate] was 2.2 mmol/l in the creatine group compared to 1.3 mmol/l for the placebo group.

Mujika et al. (1996) measured blood [lactate] and [NH_3] in 20 highly trained swimmers following 50 m and 100 m sprint swim exercise. Subjects were randomly assigned to either a placebo or creatine (20 g/d for 5 days, 100 g total) group. Blood [NH_3] after the 50 m swim decreased significantly in both groups following supplementation. Blood [NH_3] after the 100 m swim was also decreased in the creatine group, but not for the placebo group. There was no effect of creatine supplementation on blood [lactate] after either swim distance.

Kayaking Performance

In their study of kayakers, McNaughton et al. (1998) measured blood [lactate] prior to and following supplementation (20 g/day for 5 days, 100 g total) for both 90 sec and 150 sec performance test. After supplementation, post-90 sec test blood [lactate] was not significantly different from placebo and control conditions. However, post-150 sec test blood [lactate] was significantly increased following supplementation compared to placebo and control conditions. The authors concluded that the increased work accomplished during the 90 sec test without an increase in [lactate] reflected the use of the creatine supplement. The buffering capacity of creatine may explain the increased work and increased [lactate] observed during the 150 sec test following supplementation.

Chapter Summary

Improvements in performance were reported in 12 of the 22 studies presented in this chapter (mean = 16%; median = 14%). Ergogenic results are reported for laboratory-based cycle ergometry, resistive exercise, and running tasks. With one exception, the available literature is unanimous in showing no improvement in swim performance. Although more research is needed in this area, it appears that creatine supplementation may enhance performance in high-intensity tasks of more prolonged (> 30 to ≤ 150 sec) duration that rely predominantly on anaerobic glycolysis for ATP production.

7

CHAPTER

Ergogenic Effects of Creatine Supplementation on Aerobic Endurance

It has been suggested that creatine supplementation may modify substrate utilization and possibly improve performance during prolonged (> 150 sec), submaximal, steady-state (Stroud et al. 1994), or interval exercise segments incorporated into more prolonged aerobic endurance events, such as multiple periodic cycle sprints during a triathlon (Engelhardt et al. 1998). However, only limited research has been conducted in this area. This chapter reviews studies involving the effects of creatine supplementation on predominantly aerobic laboratory-based cycle ergometer and rowing tasks as well as field-based tasks such as running and swimming. Tables 7.1 to 7.3 present the key findings from these studies, with more detail as available presented in the text. Unless otherwise indicated, the studies described in this chapter employed a double-blind placebo control design. The length of the washout period is indicated for studies employing a crossover design. As in the previous chapters, *within-group* percentage changes (supplemented group or condition prescore vs. postscore) in performance (either reported by the investigators or calculated from the available data as [(post-pre)÷pre·100]) are provided. Percentage change in a repetitive exercise protocol was calculated using the pre- and postsupplementation performances for the last bout. The method of measurement of muscle [creatine] (e.g. biopsy, ^{31}P-magnetic resonance spectroscopy [^{31}P-MRS], urinary creatine/creatinine excretion) is indicated for those studies which measured creatine uptake. Studies which included biochemical markers of energy metabolism in addition to performance variables (e.g., measurement of blood [lactate], [NH$_3$], [hypoxanthinel]) will also be discussed.

Theoretically, some investigators suggest that creatine supplementation may modify substrate utilization and possibly improve performance during prolonged (> 150 sec), submaximal, steady-state or interval exercise segments incorporated into more prolonged aerobic events, such as multiple periodic cycle sprints during a triathlon.

Laboratory-Based Cycle Ergometer Exercise

Studies of the effect of creatine supplementation on aerobic cycle ergometer performance tasks are presented in table 7.1. Three studies show improved performance after creatine supplementation.

Smith et al. (1998a) randomly assigned 15 active but untrained males and females to either placebo or supplementation (20 g/day for 5 days, 100 g total). Before and after supplementation, subjects performed exercise at 3.7 W/kg body mass in addition to 5.2 W/kg anaerobic exercise, discussed in chapter 6, and 3.0 and 3.3 W/kg aerobic exercise tasks, discussed later in this chapter. Creatine ingestion resulted in a 7.2% increase in time to exhaustion at 3.7 W/kg (pre- = 236 sec; post- = 253 sec). The authors concluded that creatine supplementation improved work performance in short-duration, high-intensity aerobic exercise.

Engelhardt et al. (1998), in a preexperimental study, examined the effects of creatine supplementation (6 g/day for 5 days, 30 g total) on interval work performance within a task primarily dependent on aerobic energy production. A single-group repeated-measures design was used, and subjects were not blinded to treatments. Before and after supplementation, 12 national-class triathletes completed two consecutive periods of interval-type exercise consisting of a mean intensity of 262 W for 30 min, followed by high-intensity (anaerobic) interval exercise. The initial work rate of ~262 W elicited a blood [lactate] of ~3 mmol/L. The interval exercise was divided into two periods. Both periods included 10 intervals that were performed at 7.5 W/kg body mass for 15 sec and repeated every minute. During the intervening 45 sec, the triathletes continued to exercise at a reduced rate of 262 ± 25 W. There was a break of 120 sec between the two interval periods. Finally, the subjects repeated the endurance exercise as performed during the first 30 min of the test. Prior to supplementation, subjects completed 4.7 intervals during the first period and only 1 interval during the second period for a total of 5.7 intervals at 7.5 W/kg body mass. After supplementation, subjects increased the total number of intervals performed to 8.3 (6.3 intervals during the first period and 2 intervals during the second period). Supplementation had no effect on blood [lactate], $\dot{V}O_2$, or heart rate response. The authors concluded that 6 g of creatine/day exerted beneficial effects on intense interval exercise incorporated

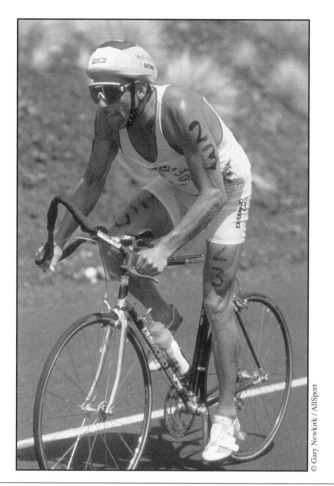

Figure 7.1 Some theorize that endurance athletes who may have repeated short bouts of high-intensity exercise in their event, such as triathletes, may benefit from creatine supplementation.

into aerobic exercise. However, they also noted that this study was a screening test and that it needs replication in a double-blind protocol.

In a study involving a clinical population, Tarnopolsky et al. (1997) gave seven male and female patients who had severe exercise intolerance both placebo and acute creatine supplementation (10 g/day for 14 days, 140 g total), followed by a maintenance regimen (4 g/day for 7 days, 28 g total). Subjects exercised on a cycle ergometer at 15 to 30 W for 5 to 10 min. Although creatine supplementation exerted no apparent effect on expired minute ventilation ($\dot{V}_E$), oxygen consumption ($\dot{V}O_2$), heart rate (HR), respiratory exchange ratio (RER), or rate of perceived exertion in comparison to the placebo treatment, the authors reported that subjects on supplementation had greater exercise tolerance.

Table 7.1 Effect of Creatine Supplementation on High-Intensity, Prolonged-Duration (> 150 sec) Cycle Ergometer Tasks Involving the Oxidative Phosphorylation Energy System.

Investigator	Year	Population	N	Gender	Design	Initial CM dose g × d = dose			Mode	Ergogenic effect?	%Δ	Comments
Engelhardt et al.	1998	Triathletes	12	M	SGRM	6	5	30	262 W for 30 min followed by 10 × 15 sec at 7.5 W/kg	Y	18	Increase in interval power performance. Possible benefit of CM on interval work incorporated into aerobic exercise training.
Smith et al.	1998a	Active untrained	15	M/F	RDBPC	20	5	100	Time to exhaustion (TTE) at 3.7 W/kg	Y	7.2	Increase in TTE from 236 sec to 253.
Tarnopolsky et al.	1997	Patients with exercise intolerance	7	M/F	RDBPCX	10 / 4	14 / 7	140 / 28	15-30 W for 5-10 min	Y	N/A	No effect on $\dot{V}_E$, RER, HR, $\dot{V}O_2$, perceived exertion.
Barnett et al.	1996	Recreationally active	17	M	RSBPC	20	6	120	$\dot{V}O_{2peak}$	N		
Godly and Yates	1997	Well-trained cyclists	16	M/F	RDBPC	20	5	100	25 km simulated race with 6 × 15 sec sprints	N		

Author	Year	Subjects	N	Sex	Design	Dose			Outcome	
Myburgh et al.	1996	Cyclists	13	M	RDBPC	20	7	140	Cycle distance in 1 hr	N
Nelson et al.	1998	Trained adults	28	M/F	SGRM	20	7-8	140-160	$\dot{V}O_{2peak}$	N
Smith et al.	1998a	Active untrained	15	M/F	RDBPC	20	5	100	Time to exhaustion at 3.3 W/kg; Time to exhaustion at 3.0 W/kg	N
Vanakoski et al.	1998	Trained athletes	7	M/F	SGRM	300 mg/kg/day	3	N/A	Aerobic exercise for 45 min.	N

RDBPC = Randomized, double-blind, placebo control

RDBPCX = Randomized, double-blind, placebo control, crossover

SGRM = Single group, repeated measures

Six studies show no improvement in aerobic cycle ergometer exercise performance after creatine supplementation. As part of a study of the effect of creatine on repetitive cycle sprint performance (described in chapter 5), Barnett et al. (1996) measured cycle ergometer $\dot{V}O_{2peak}$ in 17 recreationally active subjects before and after creatine supplementation (20 g/day for 6 days, 120 g total). Subjects were randomly assigned to either a placebo or creatine group in a double-blind manner. Creatine supplementation failed to increase $\dot{V}O_{2peak}$.

Godly and Yates (1997) measured time to completion in a simulated 25 km cycling race in which 16 well-trained male and female cyclists sprinted for 15 sec every 4 km. Subjects were randomly assigned to either placebo or creatine supplementation (20 g/day for 5 days, 100 g total). There was no significant decrease in time to completion following creatine supplementation. The authors concluded that creatine supplementation has no effect on endurance activity combined with short-duration, high-intensity bouts in well-trained subjects. These results are in contrast to those of Engelhardt et al. (1998), who reported improved performance in intense interval exercise incorporated into aerobic exercise.

Myburgh et al. (1996) assigned 13 cyclists to either a placebo or creatine (20 g/day for 7 days, 140 g total) group. Creatine supplementation increased muscle [total creatine, TCr], but did not increase the distance cycled in 1 hr.

In their study of the effect of creatine on anaerobic threshold during cycle ergometer graded exercise testing, Nelson et al. (1998) reported that maximal oxygen consumption ($\dot{V}O_{2max}$) was not increased in 28 trained adults following creatine supplementation ($\dot{V}O_{2max}$ = 3.3 1/min) compared to a nonsupplemented condition ($\dot{V}O_{2max}$ 3.4 1/min) The treatments were administered in an ordered manner, with the non-supplemented condition preceding the creatine condition. Although creatine supplementation shifted the anaerobic threshold to a higher $\dot{V}O_2$, (as discussed in chapter 6), there was no significant change in maximal aerobic power.

Smith et al. (1998a) compared the effects of creatine supplementation (20 g/day for 5 days, 100 g total) and placebo on submaximal cycle ergometer work in 15 active but untrained males and females. Dependent variables were times to exhaustion at 3.0 and 3.3 W/kg body mass. After supplementation, time to exhaustion increased by 16% (345 to 401 sec) at 3.3 W/kg and by 5% (610 to 641 sec) at 3.0 W/kg. However, these improvements were not statistically significant, presumably because of large interindividual variance.

Vanakoski et al. (1998) compared the effects of single dose of caffeine (7 mg/kg body mass), creatine (300 mg/kg body mass/day for 3 days), caffeine plus creatine, and placebo on aerobic exercise performance in seven trained athletes. Creatine uptake was confirmed by monitoring plasma [creatine] over time. Approximately 70 minutes after drug administration, subjects completed aerobic exercise on a cycle ergometer. Heart rate response was measured during exercise, but no other variables were identified in the abstract. The authors reported no significant difference in heart rate response among the four treatments. The authors concluded that aerobic performance was not significantly affected by creatine supplementation.

Of eight studies involving the effects of creatine supplementation on more prolonged aerobic cycle ergometer performance (> 150 sec), three showed an ergogenic effect on interval work performance within a task primarily dependent on aerobic energy production, an increase in time to exhaustion at 3.7 W/kg, and greater exercise tolerance in patients exercising for 5-10 min. Six studies showed no significant effects of creatine supplementation on cycle ergometer $\dot{V}O_{2peak}$, a simulated 25 km cycling race, 1 hr cycling distance, or time to exhaustion at 3.0 or 3.3 W/kg. One study reported both significant and nonsignificant ergogenic effects.

Laboratory-Based and Field-Based Running Exercise

Studies of the effect of creatine supplementation on aerobic running performance tasks are presented in table 7.2. Two field studies show increased aerobic running performance following creatine supplementation. Bocso et al. (1995) studied the effects of placebo or supplementation on the Cooper 12 min run test performance in 14 pilot cadets as well as in male soccer players. The pilot cadets were randomly assigned to either a placebo or acute supplementation (20 g/day for 5 days, 100 g total) group, and the male subjects consumed either placebo or creatine (5 g/day for 42 days, 210 g total). After supplementation, the authors reported increased distance covered during the 12 min test.

As part of their study of interval-training performance in middle distance runners, Viru et al. (1994) tested 10 trained male middle distance runners, equally assigned to either a placebo or creatine group (30 g/day for 6 days, 180 g total), on separate days before and after creatine supplementation. The tests involved 4 × 1000 m runs with 3 min recovery on separate days. The authors reported an enhanced performance in the final 1000 m run and in the total time for all 1,000 m runs. The best 1000 m run time decreased significantly by 2.1 sec (1.7%) with creatine supplementation but was unchanged by the placebo.

Two studies show laboratory and field results that fail to support the efficacy of creatine supplementation in improving aerobic running performance. Balsom et al. (1993b) randomly assigned 18 well-trained habitually active male subjects equally into either a supplementation (20 g/day for 6 days, 120 g total) or placebo group. Subjects performed a treadmill run to exhaustion at ~120% of $\dot{V}O_{2max}$ both before and after the supplementation period. Although it is reasonable to expect anaerobic glycolysis to be the predominant energy source for such a supramaximal bout, the average time to exhaustion following supplementation was reported to be 3.97 min, a performance time that appears to be more dependent on aerobic glycolysis. There

Table 7.2 Effect of Creatine Supplementation on High-Intensity, Prolonged-Duration (> 150 sec) Running Tasks Involving the Oxidative Phosphorylation Energy System.

Investigator	Year	Population	N	Gender	Design	Initial CM dose g × d = dose			Mode	Ergogenic effect?	%Δ	Comments
Bosco et al.	1995	Pilot cadets	14	M	RDBPC	20	5	100	Cooper 12 min run	Y	N/A	Increased distance run in 12 min.
Bosco et al.	1995	Soccer players	N/A	M	RDBPC	5	42	210	Cooper 12 min run	Y	N/A	
Viru et al.	1994	Middle distance runners	10	M	RSBPC	30	6	180	4 × 1,000 m interval work (85% - 90% maximal velocity)	Y	1.7	2.1 sec decrease in best 1,000 m time; improved total time for 4 × 1,000 m.
Balsom et al.	1993	Well trained	18	M	RDBPC	20	6	120	6 km terrain run time; treadmill run to exhaustion at 125% $\dot{V}O_{2max}$	N		
Stroud et al.	1994	Physically active	8	M	SGRM	20	5	100	50 - 90% $\dot{V}O_{2max}$ steady state	N		

RDBPC = Randomized, double-blind, placebo control
RSBPC = Randomized, single-blind, placebo control
SGRM = Single group, repeated measures

were no significant differences between the groups. The investigators indicated that the lack of an ergogenic effect might be expected because the energy system used would not be theorized to benefit from creatine supplementation.

Additionally, using the same supplementation protocol, Balsom et al. (1993b) had these subjects perform a 6 km terrain run on a forest trail. The authors speculated that although this type of exercise task is primarily aerobic, certain segments of the trail might stress the adenosine triphosphate-phosphocreatine (ATP-PCr) energy system. However, creatine monohydrate supplementation did not enhance performance; on the contrary, it impaired performance. The authors suggested that the impairment may have been caused by the significant gain in body mass experienced by the subjects following creatine supplementation, a finding that has also been reported by Mujika et al. (1996) in swimmers.

In order to investigate anecdotal reports of improved substrate utilization, Stroud et al. (1994) had eight men perform a continuous incremental exercise treadmill running test at various predetermined workloads approximating 50% to 90% of their $\dot{V}O_{2max}$ before and after creatine supplementation (20 g/day for 5 days, 100 g total). Subjects achieved a steady state in each protocol within 6 min, and respiratory and blood analyses both revealed that creatine supplementation did not affect energy substrate metabolism during these tests. Additionally, there were no significant effects on substrate utilization during a 15 min recovery period after the exercise bout.

Of four studies involving the effects of creatine supplementation on more prolonged aerobic running performance (> 150 sec), ergogenic effects were reported for the 12 min endurance test and for 1,000 m repeat runs. In other studies, creatine supplementation did not improve metabolic responses or endurance time in aerobic treadmill running. One study showed an impaired performance in a 6 km terrain run, presumably attributable to an increased body mass in the runners.

Miscellaneous Submaximal Exercise Performance Tasks

Three studies of the effects of creatine on miscellaneous modes of aerobic exercise (rowing, kayaking, and swimming) are presented in table 7.3. Two studies provided evidence of an ergogenic effect.

McNaughton et al. (1998) compared the effects of creatine supplementation (20 g/day for 5 days, 100 g total) and placebo on 300 sec kayak ergometer work performance in 16 elite kayakers. After creatine supplementation, there was a 6.6% (3.3 kJ) increase in work accomplished by the creatine group as compared to the placebo group.

Table 7.3 Effect of Creatine Supplementation on Miscellaneous High-Intensity, Prolonged-Duration (> 150 sec) Tasks Involving the Oxidative Phosphorylation Energy System.

Investigator	Year	Population	N	Gender	Design	Initial CM dose g × d = dose			Mode	Ergogenic effect?	%Δ	Comments
McNaughton et al.	1998	Elite kayakers	16	M	RDBPC	20	5	100	300 sec kayak work capacity	Y	6.6	3.3 kJ increase in work compared to placebo.
Rossiter et al.	1996	Rowers	38	M/F	RDBPC	20	5	100	1,000 m rowing time	Y	1.1	2.3 sec decrease in rowing time.
Thompson et al.	1996	Swimmers	10	F	RDBPC	2	42	84	400 m time	N		

RDBPC = Randomized, double-blind, placebo control

Rossiter et al. (1996) randomly assigned 38 male and female competitive rowers to either placebo or creatine-supplementation (20 g/day for 5 days, 100 g total) groups. Simulated 1,000 m rowing time was measured before and after supplementation. Total creatine uptake was estimated as the difference between creatine consumed and urinary [creatine] and [creatinine]. Muscle creatine uptake was estimated as 38 mmol/kg dry muscle. A significant 2.3 sec (1.1%) decrease in 1,000 m rowing time (211.0 to 208.7 sec) was observed in the creatine group, with no change in the placebo group. The authors also reported a trend toward significance in the association between estimated creatine uptake and percentage change in rowing performance (r = 0.43; p = 0.09).

One study, also presented in table 7.3, shows no effect of creatine supplementation on a performance task that relies primarily on aerobic metabolism. In their study on competitive female college swimmers, Thompson et al. (1996) reported that creatine supplementation (2 g/day for 56 days, 112 g total) failed to improve not only 100 m swim time, but also 400 m time.

Of three studies involving the effects of creatine supplementation on miscellaneous aerobic exercise tasks (> 150 sec), ergogenic effects were reported for 300 sec kayak ergometer and simulated 1,000 m rowing performance. No significant effects were reported for 400 m swim performance.

Performance Studies Including Biochemical Markers Reflecting Metabolic Effects of Creatine Supplementation

Cycle Ergometer Performance

Barnett et al. (1996) measured cycle ergometer $\dot{V}O_{2peak}$ in 17 recreationally active males after 6 days of either a placebo or creatine (20 g/day, 120 g total). Compared to placebo, creatine did not significantly affect blood [lactate] or pH response to exercise.

In their pre-experimental study of high-intensity interval exercise during aerobic exercise in triathletes, Engelhardt et al. (1998) reported that creatine supplementation (6 g/day for 5 days, 30 g total) had no effect on blood [lactate].

Myburgh et al. (1996) measured blood $[NH_3]$, [hypoxanthine], and [urate] during 7 days of intense sprint cycle ergometer training in 13 endurance trained cyclists assigned to either a placebo or creatine (20 g/day for 7 days, 140 g total). During the training both groups had lower $[NH_3]$ [hypoxanthine] and [urate], indicative of attenuated adenine nucleotide degradation. However, there was no difference between the groups.

Nelson et al. (1998) measured blood [lactate] and [NH$_3$] in 28 trained males and females following graded exercise testing. Subjects completed a baseline exercise test in a nonsupplemented condition, with a second test following a supplementation period (20 g/day for 7-8 days, 140-160 g total). Blood samples were obtained prior to exercise, at 6 and 12 min of exercise, at test termination, and 5 min of post exercise recovery. They reported significantly lower exercise and recovery [lactate] and [NH$_3$] following supplementation compared to baseline.

Tarnopolsky et al. (1997) studied the effect of both creatine supplementation (10 g/day for 14 days, 140 g total) and placebo on blood [lactate] response to 5-10 min of cycle ergometer exercise (15-30 watts) in seven patients with mitochondrial cytopathies. Treatment order was counterbalanced with a 5 week washout. For the creatine treatment, the authors reported a significant increase in [lactate]. Examination of their data revealed an increase from about 4.8 to 9.5 mmol/l. The authors did not indicate if the increase in blood [lactate] during exercise following the placebo treatment was significant, nor did they compare post exercise creatine and post-placebo blood [lactate].

Vanakoski et al. (1998) also measured blood [lactate] in their comparison of the effects of caffeine (a single 7 mg/kg dose), creatine (300 mg/kg body mass/day for 3 days), creatine plus caffeine, and placebo on aerobic cycle ergometer exercise. There were no differences in blood [lactate] between the four treatments.

Running Performance

Balsom et al. (1993) examined the blood [lactate] and [hypoxanthine] response to treadmill running time to exhaustion (-125% of $\dot{V}O_{2max}$) and a 6 km terrain run (~24 min) in 18 well-trained males. Subjects received either placebo or creatine supplementation (20 g/day for 6 days, 120 g total). In the creatine group, post-treadmill run blood [lactate] was significantly higher following supplementation compared to baseline. No other group or time differences in [lactate] or [hypoxanthine] were observed.

Stroud et al. (1994) examined the blood [lactate] response to steady state treadmill exercise at workrates ranging from 50 to 90% of $\dot{V}O_{2max}$ in eight physically active males prior to and following creatine supplementation (20 g/day for 5 days, 100 g total). The authors reported that creatine supplementation had no significant effect on [lactate].

Kayaking performance

McNaughton et al. (1998) examined the blood [lactate] response to a 300 sec kayak ergometer task in 16 elite male kayakers before and following creatine supplementation (20 g/day for 5 days, 100 g total). Following familiarization trials, placebo and creatine treatments were counterbalanced with a 4-week washout period. Blood [lactate] was significantly higher following supplementation compared to placebo and familiarization trials.

Isometric Exercise

Kurosawa et al. (1998a) studied the effects of creatine supplementation (30 g/day for 14 days) combined with isometric grip training on energy metabolism as measured by ^{31}P-magnetic resonance spectroscopy (^{31}P-MRS). Four males completed 2 weeks (six sessions per day) of grip exercise training consisting of 1 contraction per second to exhaustion at 30% of maximal voluntary contraction of the nondominant arm. Forearm muscle [PCr] / [β-ATP] as measured by biopsy, as well as ^{31}P-MRS, increased in both trained (21%) and untrained (11%) arms. After supplementation, muscle [PCr] depletion during exercise (20 sec) was unchanged in the trained arm (pre- 4.1 μmol; post- = 4.3 μmol) compared to the untrained arm (pre- 1.8 μmol; post- = 5.6 μmol), and muscle pH was higher in the trained arm compared to the untrained arm. These results indicate that creatine supplementation may have a negative effect on oxidative capacity in untrained skeletal muscle, but that supplementation combined with training may enhance oxidative capacity.

Summary

The studies in this section generally report no effect of creatine supplementation on such biochemical markers as [lactate], [NH$_3$], and [hypoxanthine] following prolonged (greater than 150 sec) exercise performance. In the only study reporting a lower [lactate] and [NH$_3$] response to maximal aerobic exercise (Nelson et al. 1998), the creatine treatment followed the nonsupplemented condition, thus introducing the possibility of an order effect. Two studies (Balson et al. 1993, McNaughton et al. 1998) reported a higher blood [lactate] response following creatine supplementation compared to a placebo. There appears to be little evidence that creatine modifies substrate utilization during high-intensity aerobic exercise.

Chapter Summary

Of the 16 studies discussed in this chapter, 7 support the efficacy of creatine in improving performance in tasks greater than 150 sec in duration that rely primarily on oxidative phosphorylation. Four of these studies (McNaughton et al. 1998; Rossiter et al. 1996; Smith et al. 1998a; Viru et al. 1994) show improved performance in tasks greater than 3 min in duration. These studies provide some scientific support for the concept that creatine supplementation may enhance performance in high-intensity, short-duration single or repetitive aerobic exercise tasks that may rely somewhat on anaerobic energy metabolism. There appears to be less scientific support with respect to performance tasks of longer duration that are dependent primarily on oxidative metabolism of endogenous carbohydrate and fat. This observation is probably related to relative energy system contributions with regard to aerobic performance tasks of short vs. longer duration.

8

CHAPTER

Creatine Supplementation: Effects on Body Mass and Composition

The vast majority of the human body, about 96%, consists of four elements (carbon, hydrogen, oxygen, and nitrogen) combined to form the structural basis of body protein, carbohydrate, fat, and water. The remaining 4% of our body is composed of minerals, primarily calcium and phosphorus in the bones. Because body mass and composition may exert a significant impact on health or exercise and sport performance, scientists have developed a variety of techniques to measure various body components. Currently, body composition may be evaluated at atomic, molecular, cellular, tissue-system, and whole-body levels.

Body mass represents the sum total of body materials, while body weight represents the measurement of body mass as acted upon by gravitational force. In the scientific literature of exercise and sport science, the terms body mass and body weight are often used interchangeably. The unit for mass in the Système International d'Unités (SI units) is the kilogram, which is used to represent body mass or body weight, and is easily measured with a standard medical weighing scale. In addition to body mass, of major interest to scientists in exercise and sport science are the four major components of total body mass: total body fat, fat-free mass, bone mineral content, and body water.

Total body fat consists of both essential and storage fat. Essential fat is necessary for proper functioning of certain body structures such as the brain, nerve tissue, bone marrow, and cell membranes and, in women, for reproductive purposes. Storage fat is found just under the skin (subcutaneous fat) or deep in the body, particularly in the abdominal area (visceral fat). Fat-free mass (FFM) represents the body mass devoid of all extractable fat and consisting primarily of muscle, bone, skin, organs, and water. Skeletal muscles constitute the majority of FFM. A term used inter-changeably with fat-free mass is lean body mass (LBM), but technically LBM includes essential fat. Bone consists of water, protein, and minerals, the bone mineral content representing the concentration of minerals. Water is a major constituent of all tissues, and the total body water represents both intracellular and extracellular water content.

Body mass represents the sum total of body materials, while body weight represents the measurement of body mass as acted upon by gravitational force. In the scientific literature of exercise and sport science, the terms body mass and body weight are used inter-changeably. In addition to body mass, of major interest to scientists in exercise and sport science are the four major components of total body mass: total body fat, FFM, bone mineral content, and body water.

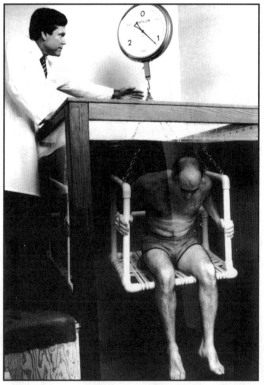

Figure 8.1 Hydrostatic, or underwater, weighing is a common technique to evaluate body composition.

Various techniques are used to evaluate body composition and to predict body fat, FFM, bone mineral content, and body water. The techniques most commonly used to determine the effect of creatine supplementation on body mass and composition include the following:

• Hydrostatic weighing: Hydrostatic, or underwater, weighing is used to determine body density based on Archimedes' principle. Various formulas are used for determination of body density, based on the gender and age of the individual. Body density is then converted to body fat and FFM.

• Skinfold measurement: The skinfold technique is designed to measure subcutaneous fat via use of skinfold calipers or ultrasound. Body fat is predicted by means of appropriate regression equations usually developed in correlation with hydrostatic weighing.

• Bioelectrical impedance analysis (BIA): Bioelectrical impedance analysis measures the resistance to a weak electrical current through the body. The greater the body water content, the lower the resistance. Based on this principle of resistance to an electrical current, BIA is used to predict body water content, body fat, and FFM.

• Dual-energy x-ray absorptiometry (DEXA): Dual-energy x-ray absorptiometry is a computerized x-ray technique used to image body tissues. By means of mathematical models, DEXA has been used to assess total body mass, body fat,

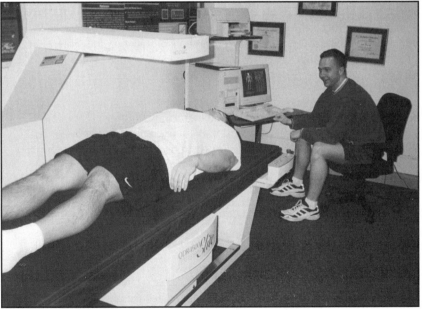

Exercise & Sport Nutrition Laboratory, University of Memphis

Figure 8.2 Dual-energy x-ray absorptiometry (DEXA) is a relatively simple, noninvasive way to evaluate body composition.

FFM, and bone mineral content, and can also assess deep visceral fat. The DEXA technique evaluates the densities of the various body components to calculate total body mass, which may be different from total body weight as measured by a weight scale.

• Magnetic resonance imaging (MRI): Magnetic resonance imaging uses magnetic-field and radio-frequency waves to image body tissues and, like DEXA, can assess deep visceral fat.

Although each of these techniques for evaluating body composition has inherent strengths and weaknesses, if applied properly each may provide useful data when one is measuring body composition changes in any given individual over time—the most common application in creatine-supplementation studies.

Creatine Supplementation and Body Mass

One of the purported effects of creatine supplementation is an increase in body mass, particularly muscle mass. As noted in chapter 3, creatine supplementation may influence body mass, and possibly body composition, in several ways. Briefly, creatine is an osmotically active substance; thus an increase in intracellular total creatine (TCr) concentration as free creatine (FCr) and phosphocreatine (PCr) may induce the influx of water into the cell, increasing intracellular water and, concomitantly, body mass (Volek et al. 1997a, 1997b; Ziegenfuss et al. 1998b). Moreover, some research suggests that increased cellular hydration and/or increased PCr may stimulate protein synthesis or decrease protein degradation, possibly increasing FFM (Clark 1997; Ingwall 1976; Volek and Kraemer 1996; Volek et al. 1997a, 1997b).

> Creatine supplementation theoretically may influence body mass, and possibly body composition, by increasing intracellular water, stimulating protein synthesis, or decreasing protein degradation.

Demographic data indicate that creatine supplementation is prevalent among individuals who desire to increase their body mass, especially muscle tissue. Many males wish to increase body mass, particularly muscle mass, for aesthetic reasons, as muscularity is a desirable masculine trait. In bodybuilding contests, a muscular somatotype is the primary determinant of successful competition. Other individuals want to increase body mass or muscle mass for competition—either to increase inertia and resist opposing forces such as those encountered in sports like sumo wrestling, or to increase muscle mass with associated gains in strength and power for sports such as competitive weight lifting. Although many nonathletes may supplement with creatine for aesthetic reasons, most athletes do so for ergogenic purposes.

> Gains in body mass, particularly muscle mass, may be ergogenic for some athletes, such as weight lifters, but detrimental to other athletes such as distance runners.

However, gains in body mass may be counterproductive for some athletes, particularly those involved in sports in which the body needs to be moved as efficiently and rapidly as possible, such as distance running. If possible gains in energy production are offset by an increased body mass, performance may not be improved and actually may be impaired. Thus for some athletes, creatine supplementation theoretically may be ergolytic.

Many studies evaluating the effect of creatine supplementation on other major dependent variables, such as muscle creatine content or various types of exercise and sport performance, also measured body mass as a minor dependent variable prior to and after supplementation. Other creatine-supplementation studies, however, have classified body mass or composition as a major dependent variable. Numerous studies have evaluated the effect of creatine supplementation on body mass—most of them looking at the short-term effects associated with 5 to 7 days of supplementation. Other studies have evaluated the effects of long-term supplementation (defined here as 14 days or longer) on body mass and composition, usually in conjunction with some form of physical training.

In this chapter we will explore the effects of creatine supplementation—both short-term and long-term—on body mass and composition in individuals varying in level of physical training. The principal details of these studies, including the citation reference, subject characteristics, experimental design, supplementation protocol, dependent variable, and results, are presented in table 8.1 for those studies showing significant increases in body mass or favorable improvement in body composition, and in table 8.2 for those studies that showed no significant changes in body mass or composition.

Short-Term Creatine Supplementation

Short-term creatine supplementation has been shown to increase body mass in diverse groups of individuals. In investigations of the effect of creatine supplementation on muscle indexes of creatine retention, such as muscle concentration of PCr, healthy, sedentary individuals often served as subjects. In other studies in which the effects of creatine supplementation on exercise or sport performance have been evaluated, several subject groups have been identified, including (a) individuals described as physically active or recreational athletes, but not highly trained; (b) highly trained athletes; and (c) resistance-trained individuals. When physically active individuals served as subjects, they often were engaging in some form of physical training.

Sedentary Subjects   Although research data are limited, several studies have shown that people need not be physically active in order to increase body mass after

Table 8.1 Creatine Supplementation: Studies Showing Significant Increases in Body Mass or Improvement of Body Composition.

Investigator	Year	Population	N	Gender	Design	Initial CM dose g × d = dose			Mode	Body changes %Δ	Comments
Balsom et al.	1995	Physically active	7	M	SGRM	20	6	120	Body mass	1.4	1.1 kg increase.
Balsom et al.	1993	Well trained	18	M	RDBPC	20	6	120	Body mass	1.2	0.9 kg increase.
Balsom et al.	1993	Active/well trained	16	M	RDBPC	25	6	150	Body mass	1.3	1.1 kg increase.
Becque et al.	1997	Weight lifters	23	M	DBPC	7	20	140	Body mass, FFM	2.3	2.0 kg increase. 1.6 kg increase.
Cooke and Barnes	1997	Healthy active	80	M	RDBPC	20	5	100	Body mass	1.2	1.0 kg increase.
Crowder et al.	1998	Lightweight football players	31	M	RDBPC	5	3	15	Body mass, skinfolds	N/A	Compared creatine powder and gum; average gain of 2.5 kg with no difference between powder and gum.
Dawson et al.	1995	Healthy active	22	M	RDBPC	20	5	100	Body mass	0.9	0.7 kg increase.
Engelhardt et al.	1998	Triathletes	12	M	SGRM	6	5	30	Body mass	N/A	0.6 kg increase.
Francaux and Poortmans	1999	Healthy, resistance training, detraining	25	M	RDBPC	21 3	5 58	105 174	Body mass	2.9	2.0 kg increase; gain may be dry matter
Goldberg and Bechtel	1997	Varsity football and track athletes	34	M	RDBPC	3	14	42	Body mass	0.9	0.9 kg increase.

Reference	Year	Subjects	N	Sex	Design				Measure	Value	Comments
Green et al.	1996a		21	M	RDBPC	20	5	100	Body mass	2	0.9 kg increase (CM) and 1.6 kg increase (CM + 500 ml CHO solution).
Green et al.	1996b	Healthy	22	M	RDBPC	20	5	100	Body mass	2.6	0.6 kg increase (CM) and 2.1 kg increase (CM + 500 ml CHO solution).
Greenhaff et al.	1994a	Healthy recreational athletes	8	M	SGRM	20	5	100	Body mass	2	1.6 kg increase.
Kelly and Jenkins	1998	Trained weight lifters	18	M	RDBPC	20	5	100	Body mass	3.2	2.8 kg increase.
Kirksey et al.	1997	Track and field athletes	36	M/F	RDBPC	20	42	840	Body mass, LBM	7.7	4.8 kg increase in LBM with CM + training compared to 3.5 kg with PL + training.
Knehans et al.	1998	Collegiate football players	25	M	RDBPC	20 / 3	5 / 60	100 / 180	FFM, total body water	4.4 / 8.2	Measured by hydrostatic weighing and bioelectrical impedance.
Kreider et al.	1998b	Football players	25	M	RDBPC	15.75	28	441	Body mass	2.5	2.42 kg increase (CM) compared to 0.85 kg (PL).
Kreider et al.	1997a	Untrained; well-trained cyclists and runners	50	M/F	RDBPC	16.5 / 15.75	14 / 14	231 / 220	Body mass, FFM	N/A	CM and Phosphagain™ both increased total body mass and FFM compared to placebo. Increase in males but not females.

(continued)

Table 8.1 *(continued)*

Investigator	Year	Population	N	Gender	Design	Initial CM dose g × d = dose			Mode	Body changes %Δ	Comments
Kreider et al.	1996a	Football players	43	M	RDBPC	20	35	700	Body mass	N/A	2.4 kg increase in LBM vs. placebo (1.04 kg).
			43	M	RDBPC	25.5	35	890	Body mass		3.45 kg increase in LBM vs. placebo (1.04 kg).
Kreider et al.	1996b	Resistance trained	28	M	RDBPC	20	28	560	Body mass	N/A	1.9 kg increase.
Maganaris and Maughan	1998	Healthy weight trained	10	M	RDBPCX	10	5	50	Body mass	2.2	1.75 kg increase.
McNaughton et al.	1998	Elite kayakers	16	M	RDBPCX	20	5	100	Body mass	2.3	1.8 kg increase.
Mihic et al.	1998	Young, healthy	30	M/F	RDBPC	20	5	100	Body mass, LBM	N/A	Increase in body mass and LBM as measured by DEXA.
Mujika et al.	1996	Swimmers	20	M/F	RDBPC	20	5	100	Body mass	1	0.7 kg increase.
Noonan et al.	1998b	College athletes	39	M	RDBPC	20	5	100	Body mass, FFM, % fat	2.58	2.7 kg increase for 300 mg/kg (25.5 g/d) group.
Ööpik et al.	1998	Karate	6	M	RDBPCX	20	5	100	Body mass	N/A	Lower loss of body mass with CM vs. placebo.

Reference	Year	Subjects	N	Sex	Design				Measure		Results
Pearson et al.	1999	Collegiate football players	16	M	RDBPC	5	70	350	Body mass, body fat	1.3	1.4 kg increase in body mass; no change in body fat as measured by skinfolds.
Peeters et al.	1999	Strength trained	35	M	RDBPC	20 / 10	3 / 39	60 / 390	Body mass, LBM	3.5	Comparison of CM vs. CP; 3.2 kg increase in LBM at 6 wk (CM).
										3	2.2 kg increase in LBM at 6 wks (CP).
Rawson et al.	1998	Older	16	M	RDBPC	20	5	100	Body mass	N/A	0.5 kg increase.
Smart et al.	1998	National soccer players	11	M	RDBPC	24	6	144	Body mass	N/A	1.9 kg increase.
Snow et al.	1998	Active untrained		M	RDBPCX	30	5	150	Body mass	1.4	1.0 kg increase.
Stone et al.	1998	Collegiate football players	9	M	RDBPC	20	35	700	Body mass, LBM	2.5 / 2.6	2.3 kg increase (measured by skinfolds and hydrostatic weighing).
Stone et al.	1999	Collegiate football players	11	M	RDBPC	8	35	280	Body mass, LBM	2.5 / 3.6	2.2 kg increase (measured by skinfolds and hydrostatic weighing).
Stroud et al.	1994	Physically active	8	M	SGRM	20	5	100	Body mass	1.3	1.0 kg increase.
Theodoru et al.	1998	Physical education students	20	M	RDBPC	25	4	100	Body mass	N/A	Increased body mass in group that ingested creatine and 500 ml of CHO vs. only creatine or placebo.

(continued)

Table 8.1 *(continued)*

Investigator	Year	Population	N	Gender	Design	g	d	dose	Mode	%Δ	Comments
Vandenberghe et al.	1997a	Healthy, sedentary	19	F	RDBPC	5	70	350	Body mass, FFM	5.8	FFM increased in both CM and PL groups at 5 wk (4.5% vs. 2.5%) and 10 wk (5.8% vs. 3.7%) training.
Viru et al.	1994	Middle distance runners	10	M	RSBPC	30	6	180	Body mass	2.5	1.8 kg increase.
Volek et al.	1999	Healthy resistance trained	25 5	M	RDBPC	7 77	175 385		Body mass FFM	2.0 6.3 2.2 6.2	1.7 kg increase in 1 wk; 5.2 kg increase in 12 wk. 1.5 kg increase in 1 wk; 4.3 kg increase in 12 wk.
Volek et al.	1997a	Healthy active	14	M	RDBPC	25	7	175	Body mass	1.8	1.4 kg increase.
Volek et al.	1997b	Normally active resistance trained	13	M	RDBPC	25	7	175	Body mass	N/A	Increase in mass due to cell hydration and a possible stimulus for anabolism.
Vukovich and Michaelis	1999	Males	48	M	RDBPC	20 10	5 16	100 160	Body mass, FFM	N/A	1.5 kg increase in body mass; 2.3 kg increase in FFM with creatine powder. 1.6 kg increase in body mass; 2.7 kg

Investigator	Year	Population	N	gender	Design	g	d	dose	Dependent variable		
Ziegenfuss et al.	1998a	Omnivorous	16	M	RDBPC	25	5	125	Body mass	1.8	increase in FFM with creatine candy.
Ziegenfuss et al.	1998b	Physically active and competitive runners	10	M	RDBPC	21	3	62	Body mass	2.0	0.86 kg increase.

Table 8.2 Creatine Supplementation: Studies Showing No Significant Changes in Body Mass or Composition.

Investigator	Year	Population	N	gender	Design	Initial CM dose g × d = dose			Dependent variable
						g	d	dose	
Barnett et al.	1996	Recreationally active	17	M	RSBPC	20	4	80	Body mass
Bermon et al.	1998	Elderly sedentary and resistance trained	32	M/F	RDBPC	20 3	5 47	100 141	Body mass
Ensign et al.	1998	U.S. Navy Seals	24	M	RDBPC	20	5	100	Body mass, %fat
Godly and Yates	1997	Well-trained cyclists	16	M/F	RDBPC	20	5	100	Body mass
Grindstaff et al.	1997	Junior competitve swimmers	18	M/F	RDBPC	21	9	189	Body mass
Hamilton-Ward et al.	1997	Athletes	20	F	RDBPC	25	7	175	Body mass
Larson et al.	1998	Soccer players	14	F	RDBPC	15	7	105	Body mass, LBM

(continued)

Table 8.2 *(continued)*

Investigator	Year	Population	N	gender	Design	Initial CM dose g × d = dose			Dependent variable
Miszko et al.	1998	NCAA IA softball players	14	F	RDBPC	25	6	150	Body mass, skinfolds
Prevost et al.	1997	Physically active college students	18	M/F	RSBPC	19	5	95	Body mass
Redondo et al.	1996	Highly trained athletes	22	M/F	RDBPC	25	7	175	Body mass
Stout et al.	1999	Football players	24	M	RDBPC	21	5	105	Body mass, FFM (DEXA)
Terrillion et al.	1997	Runners	12	F	RDBPC	20	5	100	Body mass
Theodoru et al.	1998	Physical education students	20	M	RDBPC	25	4	100	Body mass
Thompson et al.	1998	Swimmers	10	F	RDBPC	2	42	84	Body mass, LBM
Wood et al.	1998	Weight trained	44	M	RDBPC	20 2	5 37	100 34	Body mass

DBPC = Double-blind, placebo control
RDBPC = Randomized double-blind, placebo control
RCBPCX = Randomized double-blind, placebo control, crossover
SGRM = Single group, repeated measures
CHO = Carbohydrate
CM = Creatine monohydrate
CP = Creatine phosphate
PL = Placebo

short-term creatine supplementation. Ziegenfuss et al. (1998a) reported a significant average 1.8% increase in body mass in omnivorous men after creatine supplementation (0.35 g/kg body weight for 5 days). Interestingly, this effect remained for up to 28 days after cessation of creatine supplementation. Mihic et al. (1998) also reported significant increases in total body mass and LBM after creatine supplementation (20 g/day for 5 days) in healthy young males and females, but the mass changes were greater in the males than in the females. Research regarding the effects of creatine supplementation on body mass in older subjects is limited; but Rawson et al. (1998) reported a small (0.53 kg), but significant, increase in body mass after creatine loading (20 g/day for 5 days) in subjects aged 60-78 yr.

Concomitant carbohydrate intake may augment the effect of creatine supplementation on body mass. Using 21 healthy young males as subjects, Green et al. (1996a) reported that creatine loading (20 g/day for 5 days) significantly increased body mass by 0.9 kg, but that when creatine was consumed with approximately 370 g of simple carbohydrate daily, the body mass increased by 1.6 kg. However, the difference between the groups was not significant, and no data were presented to indicate any possible differences in daily energy intake associated with the additional carbohydrate.

In a follow-up study using 22 young healthy men, Green and her colleagues (1996b) reported that creatine loading increased body mass by 0.6 kg, but when an equal amount of creatine was consumed with approximately 370 g of simple carbohydrate over the course of the day, the subjects gained 2.1 kg. However, the creatine-carbohydrate group consumed approximately 3.7 mJ (880 kcal) more daily than the creatine-only group, and this may have accounted for the difference between the two groups. Additionally, carbohydrate stored as glycogen also binds water. The placebo group experienced no change in body mass. Additionally, one group of subjects consumed the creatine-carbohydrate mixture but exercised 1 hr daily at an intensity of 70% $\dot{V}O_{2max}$. For some unexplained reason, but possibly the energy expenditure or dehydration associated with the daily exercise, this group did not experience an increase in body mass.

Physically Active Individuals and Recreational Athletes   The effect of creatine supplementation on body mass has also been studied in subjects who were described as healthy and physically active or were classified as well-trained recreational athletes. Nine studies showed significant gains in body mass or body composition with creatine supplementation. Three such studies were conducted in Sweden by Balsom and his associates (Balsom et al. 1993a, 1993b, 1995). Similar creatine-supplementation protocols (20-25 g/day for 6 days) were utilized in each study, and the average gains in body mass reported for the three studies were significant, 1.1, 1.1, and 0.9 kg, while the placebo groups did not significantly increase body mass.

Dawson et al. (1995) analyzed the effect of creatine supplementation in two separate studies involving healthy, active young adult males. In one study, creatine supplementation (20 g/day for 5 days) resulted in a significant 0.7 kg gain in body mass, while the placebo group experienced a slight 0.1 kg decrease.

Greenhaff et al. (1994a) reported that creatine supplementation (20 g/day for 5 days) increased body mass by 1.6 kg in recreationally active, but not highly trained, young males. There was no control group, but seven of the eight subjects increased their body mass.

Stroud et al. (1994) reported a significant 1.0 kg body mass increase in eight physically active males after creatine loading (20 g/day for 5 days). However, the experimental protocol did not involve a control group.

Using a substantial number of healthy, active male subjects, 40 each in the creatine-supplementation group and the placebo group, Cooke and Barnes (1997) reported a significantly increased body mass averaging 1.0 kg in the creatine group, with no significant change in the placebo group.

In a double-blind, placebo crossover study, Snow et al. (1998) reported that as compared to the control trial, creatine supplementation (30 g/day for 5 days) significantly increased body mass by approximately 1 kg in active, untrained men.

Jacobs et al. (1997) investigated the effect of creatine supplementation (20 g/day for 5 days) on body mass in subjects with varied training status, some being involved in regular recreational fitness activities and others in training for competitive sports. The placebo group experienced no change in body mass following the experimental period, whereas the creatine group significantly increased body mass by 0.7 kg. Subjects ceased supplementation, and after another 7-day period the creatine group continued to maintain the weight increase.

Warber et al. (1998) reported a significant 1.5 kg (2%) increase in body mass and a 0.6% decrease in body fat in soldiers after creatine supplementation (24 g/day for 5 days), provided in sports bars. For gains in body mass associated with creatine supplementation, the form in which one consumes creatine may not matter.

In contrast to these studies presenting positive findings, four investigations showed insignificant effects of creatine supplementation on body mass. Barnett et al. (1996) reported no significant effect of creatine supplementation (20 g/day for 4 days) on body mass in recreationally active males. Although body mass tended to increase more with creatine supplementation (0.51 kg) vs. placebo (0.08 kg), the difference was not statistically significant. In the second of their studies with healthy, active young adult males, Dawson et al. (1995) reported no significant difference between the creatine-supplementation (20 g/day for 5 days) or the placebo group in body mass changes between baseline and postsupplementation trials; both groups gained about 0.5 kg.

Although they did not present body weight data, Prevost et al. (1997) reported that creatine supplementation (18.75 g/day for 5 days) had no effect on body weight in physically active young men and women. Vandenberghe et al. (1996a), using a repeated-measures crossover design with a 3-week washout period, investigated the potential ergogenic effect of creatine (0.5 g/kg for 6 days), as well as of a creatine-caffeine combination (creatine dose for 6 days, plus 5 mg/kg caffeine for 3 days), on body weight in healthy, physically active males involved in recreational sports; subjects also completed a glucose placebo trial. Although no specific body weight values were presented, the investigators did note that the body weight averaged 80 kg and did not significantly change over the three trial conditions.

Trained Athletes   Several studies have shown significant increases in the body mass of highly trained athletes after short-term creatine supplementation, even with relatively small doses of creatine.

Mujika et al. (1996) examined the effect of creatine monohydrate supplementation (20 g/day for 5 days) on the body mass of 11 male and 9 female highly trained national- and international-level competitive swimmers. Creatine supplementation was associated with a significant 0.7 kg increase in body mass, while the placebo group experienced a nonsignificant 0.3 kg decrease.

Viru et al. (1994) reported that creatine supplementation (30 g/day for 6 days) increased body weight by 1.8 kg in highly trained university middle distance runners, whereas no weight gain was reported in the placebo group.

Using 11 Bruneian national squad soccer players in the Malaysian Premier League as subjects, Smart et al. (1998) reported that creatine loading (24 g/day, with 30 g/day of glucose, for 6 days) increased body weight by 1.9 kg, whereas the placebo group maintained their body weight.

In a crossover design with a 4-week washout period, McNaughton et al. (1998), using 16 male elite surf or white-water kayak paddlers as subjects, reported a mean body mass of 77.3 kg after the creatine-supplementation (20 g/day for 5 days) phase, an increase of 2.0 kg (2.6% gain) compared to values in a placebo (75.1 kg) and two control (75.3 kg, 75.5 kg) trials. Although these investigators indicated that skinfold measurements were taken, no skinfold data were presented in the results or discussion sections.

Possibly in an attempt to gain an energy advantage associated with creatine supplementation, but also to concomitantly minimize gains in body mass that may impair performance, some athletes may consume smaller daily doses of creatine. However, Engelhardt et al. (1998) indicated that ingestion of even a low dose of creatine (6 g/day for 5 days) was associated with an increased body mass of 0.6 kg in regional-class triathletes. However, this may be considered a descriptive study as there was no control group and the authors did not indicate whether this increase was significant compared to the presupplement measurement.

Crowder et al. (1998) reported an increased body mass and decreased skinfold thickness in lightweight football players during a competitive season, including resistance training two days per week, after creatine supplementation. Two groups of subjects consumed a total of 15 g in a 3-day period, in either a powder or gum form. Dietary intake at this military academy was very well controlled. Body mass gains and skinfold thickness decreases for the powder and gum groups were, respectively, 2.3 kg, –4.5 mm and 2.7 kg, –2.6 mm, rather substantial changes in just 3 days. However, there was no real control group in this study, so the changes in body mass and composition may not be attributed to creatine supplementation. If creatine was involved in these changes, the results indicate no difference in these two forms as a means of ingesting creatine.

However, numerous other short-term studies have shown nonsignificant changes in body mass or body composition in highly trained athletes after creatine supplementation. Hamilton-Ward and her colleagues (1997) matched 20 female overhand athletes on body weight, LBM, and percent body fat and assigned them to either a placebo or creatine supplement (25 g/day) for 7 days. The creatine-supplement group gained 0.7 kg, but this increase was not significant in relation to the 0.4 kg gain in the placebo group. Terrillion and his colleagues (1997) reported no significant changes in body weight in well-trained, competitive male runners after creatine supplementation (20 g/day for 5 days), although the creatine group gained an average 0.6 kg while the placebo group lost an average 0.4 kg. Godly and Yates (1997) reported no significant effect of creatine supplementation on body mass in well-trained cyclists after creatine supplementation (20 g/day for 5 days). Studying highly trained male soccer players and female field hockey players, Redondo et al. (1996) reported no change in body weight in the placebo group, but creatine supplementation (25 g/day for 7 days) was associated with an average 0.8 kg loss in this study—one of the only studies to show a loss of body mass after creatine supplementation. The authors presented these data only for descriptive purposes and did not test the change for statistical significance.

Several studies evaluated the effect of short-term creatine supplementation on body mass and showed no significant effect.

Several investigations were designed to evaluate the effect of creatine supplementation on body composition, at least as measured by skinfold and BIA techniques. Miszko et al. (1998) examined the effect of a placebo or creatine supplement (25 g/day for 6 days) on the body mass and the sum of three skinfolds in female National Collegiate Athletic Association (NCAA) Division I softball players engaged in a standardized training routine. Although both groups gained body mass (creatine group, +1.0 kg; placebo group, +0.8 kg), there were no significant differences between or within groups pre- and postsupplementation for the sum of three skinfolds.

Ensign and associates (1998) utilized BIA to evaluate body fat and body water changes in 24 well-trained, U.S. Navy Special Warfare Seals (considered as athletes) both before and after creatine supplementation (20 g/day for 5 days). The authors reported that creatine supplementation had no significant effect on either body fat or total body water. However, whereas perusal of tabular values in this brief abstract reveals very little change in body fat in the placebo group, the body fat percentages increased a statistically nonsignificant 3.7% (12.8% to 16.5%) in the creatine-supplemented group—a rather unusual finding that might be attributed to high standard errors of measurement associated with some BIA methods.

Grindstaff et al. (1997) investigated the effect of creatine supplementation on body mass and composition of 7 male and 11 female regionally and/or nationally competitive amateur swimmers, who were matched and paired into two groups (placebo and creatine supplement) on the basis of several variables, including gender and body weight. Body mass was measured with a calibrated electronic scale (precision of ± 0.02 kg); body composition was predicted with seven-site skinfold method, and total body water was predicted by BIA. The statistical analysis revealed no significant effect of creatine supplementation (21 g/day for 9 days) on total body mass, FFM, fat mass, percent body fat, or total body water. However, because some of the probability levels approached statistical significance, the investigators suggested that 9 days of creatine supplementation may affect body composition in that changes in FFM tended to be greater and percent body fat tended to be lower in the creatine group.

Resistance-Trained Individuals   Several double-blind, placebo-controlled studies with experienced resistance-trained individuals or weight lifters also have shown positive effects of short-term creatine supplementation on body mass.

Volek et, al. (1997a), using 13 healthy, resistance-trained men as subjects, reported a significant 1.3 kg body mass increase in subjects after creatine supplementation (25 g/day for 7 days), while the placebo group experienced a nonsignificant 0.4 kg decrease in body mass. In another study using an identical experimental protocol, again with resistance-trained men but now measuring daily energy intake, Volek et al. (1997b) reported a significant 1.4 kg body mass increase associated with creatine supplementation whereas the placebo group experienced no change. The dietary analysis revealed no significant differences between the groups.

In both these reports (Volek et al. 1997a, 1997b), although they did not calculate body fat percentage, the investigators evaluated the effect of creatine supplementation on seven-site (triceps, subscapular, midaxillary, chest, suprailiac, abdomen, and thigh) skinfold thickness. There was no significant effect of creatine supplementation on the sum of the skinfold thicknesses in either study, although one of the studies showed a mean increase of 4.3 mm (Volek et al. 1997a). These findings suggest that the increase in body mass was accounted for by an increased FFM.

Maganaris and Maughan (1998), using a crossover design, reported significant increases in body mass of 10 men engaged in a weight-training program after the creatine-supplementation (10 g/day for 5 days) phase, with the first supplemented group gaining 1.7 kg and the second group, 1.8 kg. These weight gains constituted 2.3% and 2.1%, respectively, of the body mass.

In general, the vast majority of studies support the finding that short-term creatine supplementation (creatine loading) increases body mass in diverse groups of individuals including sedentary subjects, physically active individuals, recreational athletes, trained athletes, and resistance-trained individuals. In many studies showing no effect of creatine supplementation on body mass, subjects actually gained weight, but the gain was not statistically significant.

Only one study has shown no positive effect of creatine supplementation on body mass. Earnest and his colleagues (1997) found that creatine supplementation for 10 days (20 g/day for 4 days; 10 g/day for 6 days) elicited no significant changes in body weight in 14 resistance-trained individuals, including 4 runners participating in intense interval training. Although the intense running might counteract increases in body mass by consuming considerable energy, 3 of the 4 runners, by random assignment, were in the placebo group.

Short-Term Effects: Mechanisms   The gains in body mass or FFM after short-term creatine supplementation may be associated with water retention and/or increased muscle protein synthesis.

Hultman et al. (1996) reported that creatine ingestion markedly reduced urinary volume by 0.6 L during the initial days of supplementation, suggesting that the increased body mass was likely attributable to body water retention. In support of this finding, Ziegenfuss et al. (1997) reported increases of 6.6% in thigh skeletal muscle volume (measured by MRI) and 2-3% in total body and intracellular fluid volumes (measured by multifrequency BIA) in aerobic and cross-trained males after short-term creatine supplementation. In a subsequent investigation, Ziegenfuss et al. (1998b) reported a 2% increase in total body water and a 3% increase in intracellular water, with no change in extracellular water, after 3 days of creatine supplementation (0.35 g/kg FFM per day). The findings, the authors noted, seemed to indicate that weight gain associated with short-term creatine supplementation is primarily a result of water retention, mostly within the intracellular compartment.

During the short-term loading protocol, approximately 30-40 g of creatine is retained in the body, yet subjects reportedly gain 0.5 to 1.0 kg body mass. Even when using the lowest retention amount (30 g) and the lowest weight gain (0.5 kg, or 500 ml water), each gram of creatine would have to cause the retention of approximately 15 ml, or grams, of water. Muscle creatine uptake is sodium dependent, so if sodium concentration increases intracellularly, its osmotic properties could increase fluid retention.

Another possibility may be increased protein synthesis. Ziegenfuss and his colleagues (1997) reported preliminary evidence of improved nitrogen status (decreased degradation and/or increased synthesis as measured by ^{15}N-glycine tracer) in experienced weight lifters after short-term creatine supplementation. Since muscle is composed of approximately 22% protein, with the remainder mostly water, protein synthesis would have to produce only about 22% of the weight gain, or about 110 g of protein for a 0.5 kg gain over 3 days—an average of about 35 g protein synthesis per day. Each gram of protein would bind about 3-4 g of water. For an 80 kg athlete with 35 kg muscle mass, this would be only about 1 g of protein synthesis per kilogram muscle mass daily, which is not much considering normal daily turnover. However, research is needed to document this speculation.

Most research findings suggest that the gains in body mass after short-term creatine supplementation may be associated with water retention, although one study provided evidence of improved nitrogen (protein) status.

Long-Term Creatine Supplementation

Several earlier clinical investigations involving long-term creatine or creatine phosphate supplementation to patients with various medical problems revealed some interesting data regarding body mass. Sipilä et al. (1981), treating patients who had gyrate atrophy with 1.5 g of creatine per day for a year, reported an approximate 10% gain in body weight at the start of the treatment; but then the weight remained stable. Additionally, the authors reported a reversal of the type II muscle fiber atrophy associated with this disease, noting a 42% increase in type II muscle fiber diameter. Pirola and associates (1991) investigated the effect of intramuscular injections of PCr, 500 mg daily for 20 days, as an adjunct to a physiokinesitherapy rehabilitation program for patients who had muscle hypotrophy of the lower limbs due to fracture of the thigh. The PCr group had an increase in muscle mass of 4.4 mm, as determined by echotomography, while the group receiving only physiokinesitherapy increased muscle mass by only 1.5 mm; the difference between the groups was statistically significant.

Although some research has been conducted with sedentary individuals undertaking physical training, most experimental long-term creatine-supplementation studies addressing an ergogenic effect on body mass or composition have been conducted with physically active individuals or athletes who were usually involved in some form of training, either resistance training or training specific to their sport. Most, but not all, long-term supplementation studies incorporated a loading phase followed by a longer maintenance phase. Studies lasting 14 days or longer are classified as long-term.

Research Supporting a Beneficial Effect   Resistance training is an effective means to increase body mass and FFM, and some research has shown that creatine supplementation may augment this effect—not only in untrained individuals but in highly trained people as well. The following studies are presented in order of length of the supplementation period.

Kreider et al. (1996a) evaluated the effects of two commercial dietary supplements containing slightly different amounts of creatine (Phosphagain™, 20 g/day; Phosphagain II™, 25.5 g/day) on development of lean tissue mass in 42 NCAA Division IA football players undergoing 35 days of off-season resistance and agility training. Each supplement contained various amounts of other nutrients and dietary components. Gains in lean tissue mass, measured by DEXA, were significantly greater in the Phosphagain™ and Phosphagain II™ groups (2.43 and 3.45 kg, respectively) compared to the placebo group (1.04 kg), but there was no significant difference between the two commercial supplements.

Earnest et al. (1995) reported a significant 1.7 kg increase in the body mass of experienced weight-trained males after creatine loading (20 g/day for 14 days). The placebo group experienced no significant changes.

Evaluating possible different responses in untrained vs. trained subjects, Kreider et al. (1997a) investigated the effect of creatine supplementation on body mass, total body water, and body composition (measured by BIA and skinfolds) in 24 untrained males and females and 26 well-trained cyclists and runners. Subjects were matched on training status and body mass and were assigned to one of three groups: placebo, creatine (16.5 g/day), or a commercial product (Phosphagen HP™) containing primarily creatine and glucose (15.75 g/day and 99 g/day, respectively) for 14 days. Gains in body mass and FFM tended to be greater, but not statistically significant (p = 0.10), in the two creatine groups compared to the placebo group. When the two creatine groups were combined and compared to the placebo group, significant differences were observed in total body mass (0.94 vs. 0.23 kg gain) and FFM (0.87 vs. 0.20 kg). No significant differences were observed among groups in total body water, fat mass, or percent body fat. Furthermore, no differences were seen between trained and untrained groups. Gender analysis revealed that creatine and Phosphagen HP™ promoted significant increases in total body mass and FFM in males but had no effects in females.

Kelly and Jenkins (1998) investigated the effect of a long-term 26-day creatine-supplementation protocol (20 g/day for 5 days; 5 g/day for the next 21 days) on body mass and composition in trained power lifters. Body composition was predicted from skinfold measurements. Creatine supplementation significantly increased body mass by an average of 2.8 kg (88.8 to 91.6 kg) over the 26-day period, whereas no significant changes were observed in the placebo group. The authors also evaluated daily energy intake, noting that it was unlikely that differences in energy intake caused the large increase in body mass in the creatine group. There was no significant change in percent body fat in either group, but the significant increase in LBM after creatine supplementation was comparable to the increase in body mass. As noted in chapter 5, the creatine-supplement group experienced significant gains in bench press strength and repetitions, and these gains were associated with the gains in body mass—both in absolute terms and relative to body mass.

Some studies have addressed the effect on body composition of various dietary supplements designed to promote lean tissue accretion. Numerous nutrients have been theorized to be anabolic, including amino acids such as arginine and ornithine and minerals such as boron, chromium, and vanadium. Creatine monohydrate, a component of some of these commercial products, has been compared to other such products in several investigations. For example, Kreider et al. (1996b) compared the effects of a creatine-containing commercial product, as contrasted to a maltodextrin placebo and another creatine-free commercial product, on body mass and composition changes in 28 resistance-trained males over a 28-day period. The creatine dosage was 20 g/day for 28 days. Body weight significantly improved in all three groups. Total body mass as scanned by DEXA also increased significantly in all three groups, but significantly greater gains were reported for the two commercial supplement groups. Moreover, lean tissue mass (excluding bone) gain was greater in the creatine group.

In a later study, Kreider et al. (1998b) examined the effect of creatine supplementation (15.75 g/day for 28 days) on body mass and composition in 25 NCAA Division I football players engaged in resistance/agility training for 8 hr per week. Subjects were matched by total body weight and assigned to the creatine (added to commercial product) or placebo (commercial product only) group. Nutritional intake was monitored before and near the completion of the study. Total body weight was measured on a calibrated digital scale with a precision of ± 0.02 kg, and body composition was determined by DEXA. Total body weight increased significantly in both groups, but gains were significantly greater in the creatine group. The creatine group gained 2.42 kg, and the placebo group gained 0.85 kg. No significant differences were observed between groups in total body water changes expressed as a percentage of total body weight; this suggested that changes were not attributable to body water changes. There were no significant differences between groups in the mean estimated total daily energy intake, suggesting that energy intake differences did not account for the body mass difference between groups. Also, no significant differences were observed in mean changes in bone mass, fat mass, or percent body fat between the groups. However, DEXA-scanned total body mass and fat/bone-free mass were significantly increased in the creatine group. But as the investigators note in both this study and the earlier one (Kreider et al. 1996b), since many commercial products contain a number of nutrients it is unclear which nutrient or combination of nutrients may elicit anabolic effects. Although the effects on body mass or composition in this study might be attributable to creatine (because the commercial product served as the placebo), some interactions between the nutrients in the product and creatine might occur that could affect body mass or composition.

In a 2×2 factorial design, Stone et al. (1999) evaluated the effect of creatine supplementation, with and without pyruvate, on body mass and body composition in NCAA Division IAA football players engaged in physical training, including resistance training. Subjects in the supplement groups consumed 0.22 g/kg per day of their specific supplement. For the creatine-only group, the total creatine was 0.22 g/kg per day, but for the creatine-pyruvate group it was only 0.09 g/kg per day; the daily total creatine intake for these two groups approximated 20 and 8 g, respectively. The supplementation period was 5 weeks. Body mass and LBM, as measured by both hydrostatic weighing and skinfolds, increased significantly more in both the creatine groups compared to the placebo and pyruvate-only groups. The average body mass gain in each creatine group was about 2.3 kg, a 2.5% change; the percentage gains in LBM were even greater, as the subjects also lost body fat.

Becque et al. (1997) reported that creatine supplementation for 6 weeks (20 g/day for 7 days, 2 g/day for 5 weeks) significantly increased both body mass (2.0 kg) and FFM (1.6 kg) during a strength-training regimen, while there were no changes in the placebo group. Additionally, there were no changes in body fat mass or percent body fat in either group. Hydrostatic techniques were used to evaluate body composition.

Peeters et al. (1999) compared the effects of two forms of creatine (creatine monohydrate and creatine phosphate), as compared to a placebo, on body composition in 35 strength-trained males (2 years experience). The 6-week study involved both a creatine-loading phase (20 g/day for 3 days) and a maintenance phase (10 g/day through 6 weeks). Body composition was predicted by the skinfold technique. After 3 weeks, both creatine groups significantly increased LBM compared to the placebo group, and these increases were maintained during the subsequent 3 weeks of supplementation. There were no significant differences between the creatine groups. The pretest, post-3 week, and post-6 week LBM values for the creatine monohydrate group were 76.7, 80.0, and 79.9 kg, respectively, and the corresponding values for the creatine phosphate group were 73.5, 74.2, and 75.7 kg; the placebo group values were 75.3, 75.5, and 75.4 kg.

In both male and female track and field athletes undergoing preseason conditioning, Kirksey et al. (1997) reported a 4.8 kg increase in LBM, as estimated by skinfold measurements, after 6 weeks of creatine supplementation (0.3 g/kg per day [i.e., ~20 g/day]). However, an increase of 3.5 kg in LBM attributed to physical training was also observed in the placebo group.

Over the course of 8 weeks, Stout and colleagues (1999) evaluated the effects of creatine supplementation on LBM in NCAA Division II football players engaged in resistance training and speed drills 4 days per week. Three groups of subjects consumed either a placebo, creatine monohydrate, or a commercial supplement containing creatine monohydrate plus glucose, taurine, and sodium and potassium phosphates. The creatine dosage in both creatine groups was 21 g/day for 5 days and 10.5 g/day for the remainder of the 8 weeks. Fat-free mass was measured by DEXA. The placebo group lost 0.01 kg FFM, whereas the creatine and commercial creatine product groups gained, respectively, 2.6 and 2.9 kg FFM. However, although the gains in FFM for the group consuming the commercial product were significantly greater than those for the placebo group, the gains for the creatine group, although substantial, were not.

Noonan et al. (1998b) studied the effect of 8-week creatine supplementation on body mass and body composition in 39 college athletes divided into three equal groups, one receiving a placebo and the other two receiving varying dosages of creatine based on body mass. After a creatine-loading phase (20 g/day for 5 days), for the remainder of the 8 weeks two groups received a daily maintenance dose of creatine standardized on FFM; one group received 100 mg/kg FFM, and the other group received 300 mg/kg FFM. These doses were designed to replicate the lowest and highest dosages cited in the scientific literature as improving exercise performance. The athletes were involved in a conditioning program four times per week that emphasized weight training and speed drills. Body weight was measured on a medical-grade scale accurate to the nearest 100 g, while body composition was determined by hydrostatic techniques. The overall statistical analysis revealed no significant differences among any of three groups for body mass, percent body fat, or FFM, although the overall F ratio approached statistical significance. Conducting a within-group statistical analysis, the investigators found that the placebo group had gained 0.37% body mass, a nonsignificant increase. The 100 mg group had gained 2.87% body mass, which was not significant, whereas the 300 mg group had gained 2.55% body mass—a significant gain even though it was less than the absolute gain in the 100 mg group. The FFM for the placebo, 100 mg, and 300 mg groups increased, respectively, 1.80%, 3.73%, and 2.58%, and the within-group statistical analysis revealed that the FFM increases in the 100 mg and 300 mg groups were significant. Interestingly, the control group was the only group to significantly reduce body fat as revealed by the within-group analysis.

In a 9-week study, Knehans et al. (1998) investigated the effect of creatine supplementation (20 g/day for 5 days, followed by 3 g/day for the remainder of the 9 weeks) on body composition in university football players involved in a supervised weight-training program. Using hydrostatic weighing and BIA, they reported significant increases in LBM (4.4%), total body water (5%), and intracellular water (8.2%) in the creatine group, with no significant changes in the placebo group.

Francaux and Poortmans (1999) assigned 25 healthy male subjects to either a control, placebo, or creatine (21 g/day for 5 days; 3 g/day for next 58 days) group, with the placebo and creatine groups participating in a 9-week program that included resistance training for 42 days followed by a detraining period of 21 days. No change in body mass was oserved in the control and placebo groups during the entire experimental period, while body mass in the creatine group significantly increased by 2 kg, a 2.9% increase. Using bio-impedance spectroscopy, the increased body mass was attributed partially to an increase in total body water content, more specifically to an increase in the volume of the intracellular compartment. Nevertheless, these investigators concluded that the relative volumes of body water compartments remained constant and therefore the gain in body mass cannot be attributed to water retention, but probably to dry matter growth accompanied with a normal water volume.

Vandenberghe et al. (1997a) studied the effect of 4 days of high-dose (20 g/day) followed by 10 weeks of low-dose (5 g/day) creatine supplementation on body mass and composition of 19 sedentary young adult females initiating a resistance-training program. Body composition was assessed by the hydrostatic weighing method. There were no significant differences in body mass between the groups, the placebo group gaining an average of 1.0 kg and the creatine group, 1.8 kg. Body fat tended to decrease during the training plus low-dose period, but these changes were not significantly different between the two groups. However, the gains in LBM in the creatine group (2.6 kg) were significantly greater than those in the placebo group (1.6 kg). Compared with initial values, percentage gains in FFM increased significantly more in the creatine group than in the placebo group after both 5 (creatine group, 4.5%; placebo group, 2.5%) and 10 weeks (creatine group 5.8% to placebo group 3.7%). According to the investigators, the data presented clearly demonstrate that long-term creatine supplementation increases total body FFM.

Using a randomized, double-blind protocol, Volek et al. (1999) evaluated the effect of creatine supplementation (25 g/day for 7 days; 5 g/day for 11 weeks) on body mass and body composition (determined by hydrostatic weighing) in 19 resistance-trained men undergoing periodized heavy resistance training three to four times per week for 12 weeks. Muscle biopsies were also taken prior to, after 1 week, and after the 12-week training program to evaluate muscle fiber changes. After 1 week, body mass (82.1 to 83.8 kg) and FFM (68.7 to 70.2 kg) were significantly elevated in the creatine group, but not the placebo group; after 12 weeks, both groups significantly increased body mass (creatine, 82.1 to 87.3 kg;

placebo, 82.9 to 85.9 kg) and FFM (creatine 68.7 to 73.0 kg; placebo, 68.6 to 70.7 kg), but the increases were significantly greater in the creatine subjects. Additionally, creatine subjects demonstrated significantly greater increases in type I, IIA, and IIAB muscle fiber cross sectional areas at 12 weeks. These investigators concluded that creatine supplementation increased body mass and enhanced FFM and muscle morphology.

Investigations on the effects of long-term (2-12 weeks) creatine supplementation on body mass and composition have been conducted primarily with physically active individuals or athletes who are usually involved in some form of training—either resistance training or training specific to their sport. Of nearly 20 studies, about 80% showed significant gains in either body mass or various measures of FFM after creatine supplementation. Even in those studies showing no effects, creatine supplementation induced gains in body mass or FFM, but the gains were not statistically significant.

Research Showing No Beneficial Effects   Several studies have not shown any additive effects of creatine supplementation on body mass or composition in comparison to those attributable to resistance training or other forms of training.

Earnest et al. (1995) reported a nonsignificant 1.6 kg increase in the calculated FFM of experienced weight-trained males after creatine loading (20 g/day for 14 days). In this study, as noted earlier, the increase in total body mass was 1.7 kg, which was a significant change. This 1.6 kg increase in FFM indicates that almost all the 1.7 kg gain in body mass was accounted for by an increased FFM; nevertheless, this gain in FFM was statistically nonsignificant, although the reported probability value was 0.054. The placebo group experienced no significant changes. Body composition was measured by hydrostatic procedures.

Using a factorial, double-blind, placebo research design, Bermon et al. (1998) reported no significant effect of creatine supplementation (20 g/day for 5 days; 3 g/day for 47 days) on body mass, body fat (skinfolds), and lower limb muscular volume (estimated from skinfolds/circumferences) in sedentary, elderly (67-80 years) men and women who either remained sedentary or engaged in 8 weeks of resistance training.

Wood et al. (1998), using 44 resistance-trained college males who trained at least once weekly, reported that 6 weeks of creatine supplementation (20 g/day for 5 days; 2 g/day for 37 days) had no significant effect on lean body mass, as measured by hydrostatic weighing, or on chest, abdominal, thigh, or arm girths.

Thompson et al. (1996) reported no significant changes in LBM of female nonvegetarian swimmers after prolonged creatine supplementation (6 weeks), albeit with a small dose (2 g/day). No LBM data were presented, nor was the method of evaluating LBM identified, although the investigators did use magnetic resonance spectroscopy to examine muscle concentrations of creatine. Also using females as subjects, Larson et al. (1998) evaluated the effect of creatine supplementation or a placebo on body composition changes of university female soccer players over the course of 13 weeks of training. The creatine-loading dose was 15 g/day for 1 week, followed by a maintenance dose of 5 g/day thereafter. As measured by DEXA, the placebo group gained 1.02 kg LBM, while the creatine group gained 1.83 kg; however, there was no statistically significant difference between the groups.

Long-Term Effects: Mechanisms   These studies suggest that creatine supplementation augments increases in body weight and FFM normally associated with resistance training. If creatine enables individuals to train more intensely, then part of the increase in FFM could be muscle tissue. However, according to Vandenberghe et al. (1997a), although the data presented in their study clearly demonstrate that long-term creatine supplementation increases body FFM, it must be emphasized that the increase in FFM may at least partly result from increased muscle water content. Nevertheless, data from Francaux and Poortmans (1999) suggests much of the increase is dry matter.

If creatine enables individuals to train more intensely, then part of the increase in FFM could be muscle tissue. Some investigators hypothesize that an increased cellular hydration induced by creatine supplementation may increase protein synthesis and decrease protein degradation, and several studies have reported significantly increased muscle mass after the long-term creatine supplementation. However, confirming research is recommended.

As discussed in chapter 3, an increased cellular hydration induced by creatine supplementation may increase protein synthesis, decrease protein degradation, and thus increase FFM (Häussinger et al. 1993; Volek et al. 1997a, 1997b). Ziegenfuss et al. (1998b), using multifrequency BIA, recently reported that the first 3 days of creatine loading induces an increase in intracellular fluid with no change in extracellular fluid. Theoretically, this increased intracellular fluid may stimulate protein synthesis over time. Additionally, Kreider et al. (1998b) reported similar effects, noting that the ratio of urea nitrogen to creatinine was decreased in athletes ingesting creatine during intense resistance/agility training.

Creatine Supplementation During Weight Loss

Athletes in weight-control sports, such as wrestling, boxing, and karate, attempt to lose body mass in order to compete at an optimal body weight classification. However, they also want to maintain muscle mass and muscular strength and endurance, which are purported ergogenic benefits of creatine supplementation. On the other hand, if creatine leads to increased body mass, supplementation may be counterproductive to achieving an optimal weight class. To explore this issue, Ööpik and his colleagues (1998) evaluated the effect of creatine supplementation in six well-trained male karate athletes who were experienced in weight-loss practices in preparation for competition. In this repeated-measures, crossover design with a 1-month washout period, subjects consumed either a glucose placebo or 20 g of creatine monohydrate daily for 5 days during a period of body mass reduction. The subjects were asked to reduce their body mass by 5% over the 5 days, using whatever techniques they normally did but not using pharmacological agents. Subjects also kept a detailed record of diet and physical activity. The same weight-loss techniques were used during both trials. The extent of body mass loss in the placebo trial was significantly greater than in the creatine trial: 3.3 kg (4.3%) vs. 2.2 kg (3.0%), respectively. As there were no differences in the energy intake between the placebo and creatine trials on any of the 5 days, the investigators contend that creatine supplementation reduced the efficacy of energy restriction and other methods used for body mass reduction. However, in the creatine condition the athletes were at a lower weight at the beginning of the restriction period, which could have influenced their ability to lose weight. For the placebo trial the weights were 76.1 kg before and 72.8 kg after, and for the creatine trial the weights were 74.4 kg before and 72.1 kg after.

For athletes in weight-control sports such as wrestling, boxing, and karate, creatine supplementation may impair attempts to lose body mass in order to compete at an optimal body weight classification.

As noted in chapter 6, contrary to expectations, the normal negative influence of body mass reduction on submaximal physical working capacity was not reduced but in fact was amplified by the creatine treatment. The body mass reduction caused an approximately twofold decrease in plasma volume in the creatine trial in comparison to the placebo trial; but the difference was not significant, and the investigators noted that the extent of the relative decrease in plasma volume was small in both trials, suggesting that changes in plasma volume did not explain this decrease in submaximal exercise performance. The authors speculated that muscle creatine uptake could have been impaired because of inadequate carbohydrate intake during body mass loss, or that creatine consumed by highly trained strength and power athletes in order to improve their working capacity may be considerably less efficient than in the case of nontrained subjects. Another possibility is a type I statistical error, as multiple paired-sample t-tests were used to test differences within each trial, not between the treatments. The graphical description of the curves for submaximal work look similar for placebo and creatine; the difference is within the creatine group, that is, before and after, not between the creatine and placebo trials, where graphically the creatine group actually looks to have performed better. This is an important area of research in which replication studies are needed.

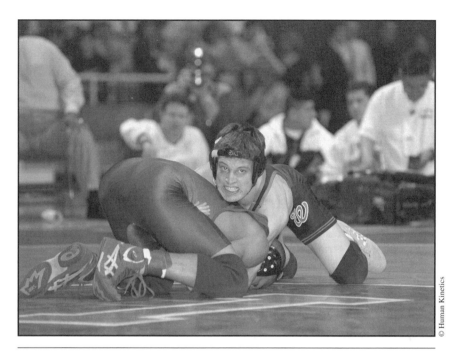

Figure 8.3   Creatine supplementation may hinder weight loss in weight-control sports such as wrestling.

Possible Ergolytic Effects

Some investigators suggest that increased body weight may be ergolytic for some athletes. An increased body mass, without enhancement of energy efficiency, could impair performance in exercise or sport tasks dependent on moving the body mass from one point to another in an efficient manner. For example, Mujika et al. (1996) suggested that the increased body weight associated with creatine supplementation may increase hydrostatic drag and therefore contribute to slower swim sprint times, while the results of the study by Miszko et al. (1998), although not conclusive, suggest that a creatine-loading weight gain might impair vertical jump performance. Balsom and his colleagues (1993b) also suggest that a significant weight gain could impair endurance running performance.

> In some athletes, a creatine supplementation-induced increase in body mass without enhancement of energy efficiency could impair performance in exercise or sport tasks dependent on moving the body mass from one point to another in an efficient manner, such as distance running.

However, with the exception of the study of Balsom et al. (1993b), who reported an impaired performance in a 6 km terrain run on a forest trail after creatine supplementation, studies have normally not shown impaired exercise or sport performances in situations in which the body is moved—although most also do not show a beneficial ergogenic effect. For example, as already noted, Smart et al. (1998) reported a 1.9 kg increase in body mass in Bruneian national squad soccer players after 1 week of creatine loading, while the placebo group maintained their weight. The players were also tested in repeat running sprints, as discussed in chapter 5, and creatine supplementation did not increase speed. These investigators suggested that this finding may have been influenced by the increase in body mass in the creatine-supplemented players. Although the creatine-supplemented players did not improve speed, their weight gain did not significantly impair performance—suggesting that creatine supplementation was not ergolytic, but rather neutral, relative to repetitive sprint performance. For some athletes, an increased body mass with no speed impairment may be advantageous. Moreover, a recent study documented increased speed in the first three of eight 40-m sprints after creatine supplementation.

Chapter Summary

Overall, it would appear that short-term creatine supplementation may contribute to increased total body mass, at least in males, although much of the increase in body mass may be attributed to water retention rather than increased contractile protein. Chronic creatine supplementation, combined with resistance training, may increase LBM, but more supportive research is desirable to determine efficacy and the possible underlying mechanism.

Kreider et al. (1998b) recommend additional research to evaluate the effects of creatine supplementation on body composition, on fluid retention and total body water content with use of more precise methods, and on protein synthesis, including any potential additive or synergistic effects that substances in commercial products may have on lean tissue accretion during training.

"When I'm taking creatine it helps me retain my strength and size, and my energy level is a lot better."

Greg Foster, Utah Jazz Center
Strauss, G., and Mihoces, G. (1998).

9

Health and Safety Aspects of Creatine Supplementation

Although anecdotal reports indicate that elite athletes have been supplementing their diets with creatine since the 1960s (Gola 1998; Plisk and Kreider 1999), widespread use of creatine as a nutritional supplement did not occur until the early 1990s when synthetic creatine began to be marketed by nutritional supplement companies. Likewise, although research on the metabolic and therapeutic role of creatine has been conducted for some time, the majority of studies addressing the ergogenic value of creatine supplementation in athletes did not begin until the early to mid-1990s. Given that widespread creatine use among athletes is a relatively new phenomenon, concern has been raised regarding the health risks associated with creatine supplementation. The intent of this chapter is to evaluate the available evidence regarding the clinical effects, medical uses, and anecdotally reported side effects of creatine supplementation in nonathletic, athletic, and diseased populations.

Effects of Creatine Supplementation on Markers of Clinical Status

Several groups of researchers have investigated the effects of creatine and phosphocreatine (PCr) supplementation (oral or injectable) on various markers of clinical status. These reports provide valuable insights as to the medical safety of creatine supplementation. In this section we describe some of the reported effects of creatine supplementation on endogenous creatine synthesis, renal function, muscle and liver enzyme efflux, blood volume and electrolytes, blood pressure, and lipid profiles.

Given the fact that widespread creatine use among athletes is a relatively new phenomenon, concern has been raised regarding the health risks associated with creatine supplementation.

Endogenous Creatine Synthesis

When exogenous intake of creatine is increased (through the diet or supplementation), animal studies indicate that endogenous creatine synthesis is temporarily suppressed (Guerrero-Ontiveros and Wallimann 1998). Consequently, some concern has been raised about whether long-term creatine supplementation may permanently suppress endogenous creatine synthesis. Although long-term data are limited, several studies have evaluated the effects of cessation of short- and long-term creatine supplementation on muscle total creatine (TCr) and PCr levels and provide some insight. In this regard, studies have shown that it takes about 4 to 5 weeks after cessation of short- or long-term creatine supplementation for elevated muscle TCr and PCr levels to return to normal (Febbraio et al. 1995; Hultman et al. 1996; Lemon et al. 1995; Vandenberghe et al. 1997a).

For example, Lemon et al. (1995) reported that one subject still had significantly higher muscle PCr levels 5 weeks after cessation of creatine supplementation (20 g/day for 5 days). Additionally, Vandenberghe and coworkers (1997a) reported that after 4-week cessation of creatine supplementation (20 g/day for 4 days followed by 5 g/day for 136 days), muscle PCr levels returned toward baseline but were still higher than presupplementation values.

Endogenous synthesis of creatine accounts for about 1 g/day of the daily creatine requirement (see chapter 2). Therefore, if creatine supplementation permanently suppressed endogenous creatine synthesis, one would expect muscle TCr and PCr levels to fall well below baseline after 4 to 5 weeks of cessation of creatine supplementation. Moreover, since creatine deficiency has been reported to be associated with fatigue, muscle atrophy, poor exercise capacity, and/or neuromuscular deficiencies, it could be argued that if creatine supplementation resulted in long-term suppression of creatine synthesis, former creatine users would present with some of these symptoms. Although additional research is needed, there is currently no evidence that creatine supplementation causes a long-term suppression of creatine synthesis.

Although creatine supplementation may suppress endogenous creatine synthesis during supplementation, there is currently no evidence that creatine supplementation causes a long-term suppression of creatine synthesis after cessation of supplementation.

Renal Function

As described in chapter 3, when creatine is ingested, serum creatine levels typically increase for several hours. Creatine storage into the muscle primarily occurs during the first several days of creatine supplementation. Thereafter, excess creatine that is ingested is primarily excreted as creatine in the urine, with a small amount of creatine converted to creatinine in the muscle (Chanutin 1926; Crim et al. 1975, 1976; Poortmans et al. 1997; Vandenberghe et al. 1997a).

Large increases in serum and urinary creatinine (up to 10-fold) have been used clinically as a basic indicator of tissue degradation and/or kidney stress. However, intense exercise and dehydration can also serve to increase serum and urinary creatinine excretion (Janssen et al. 1989; Irving et al. 1986, 1990; Kargotich et al. 1997; Long et al. 1990). Serum and urinary creatinine levels have been reported to be either not affected or slightly increased following creatine supplementation (Crim et al. 1975, 1976; Earnest et al. 1996a, 1996b; Engelhardt et al. 1998; Kreider et al. 1998b, 1999b; Poortmans et al. 1997; Sipilä et al. 1981; Vandenberghe et al. 1997a). It has been suggested that the increased serum and urinary creatinine levels reflect an increased release and cycling of intramuscular creatine as a consequence of enhanced muscle protein turnover and/or greater training volume in response to creatine supplementation and not a pathologic origin (Balsom et al. 1994; Chanutin 1926; Earnest et al. 1996b; Harris et al. 1992; Kreider et al. 1998b; Poortmans et al. 1997; Vandenberghe et al. 1997a).

However, others contend that the elevations in serum and urinary creatinine after creatine supplementation as reported in some studies may be indicative of greater renal stress. To support this view, two recent case-study reports have suggested that elevations in serum creatinine in an asthmatic athlete during two-a-day football practices (Kuehl et al. 1998), and in a patient with preexisting renal disease (Pritchard and Kaira 1998) who reported taking creatine, represented evidence of renal stress. Although the conclusions of these reports have been criticized (Greenhaff 1998; Poortmans and Francaux 1998), the possibility that creatine supplementation may increase renal stress cannot be completely discounted in that few short- or long-term studies have evaluated the effects of creatine supplementation on renal function. In the following paragraphs we describe results from available studies.

Poortmans et al. (1997) investigated the effects of creatine supplementation (20 g/day for 5 days) on renal responses in healthy men. The researchers found that after creatine supplementation, arterial creatine content, urinary creatine content, and creatine clearance were significantly increased (2.7-, 89-, and 26-fold increase, respectively). However, although increased slightly, no significant differences were seen in arterial creatinine levels, urinary creatinine levels, or 24 hr creatinine clearance (8.3%, 6.6%, and 3.8%, respectively). This latter observation is important in that marked elevation in creatinine clearance serves as a clinical marker of renal stress. In a separate paper, Poortmans and Francaux (1998) reported that creatine supplementation (20 g/day for 5 days, 3 g/day thereafter) did not significantly affect creatinine clearance, urea clearance, or albumin clearance after 5, 20, 41, and 63 days of supplementation. These findings indicate that excess creatine is excreted in the urine without a significant amount being converted to creatinine. The results further indicate that there is no evidence of increased renal stress during supplementation trials lasting up to 9 weeks as determined by creatinine clearance studies.

Engelhardt and colleagues (1998) evaluated the effects of creatine supplementation (6 g/day for 5 days) on pre- and postexercise creatine and creatinine concentrations in the blood and urine. The researchers reported that creatine supplementation increased preexercise serum creatine by 50% (74.3 to 111.7 μmol/L) and creatinine levels by 16.3% (62.7 to 79 μmol/L). Moreover, pre- and postexercise urine excretion of creatine was increased by 1,400% (0.22 to 3.1 mmol/L) while creatinine levels were increased by 66% (9.2 to 15.3 mmol/L). These findings support contentions that excess creatine is primarily excreted as creatine in the urine and that serum and urinary creatinine levels may be increased in response to creatine supplementation. However, it is unclear whether these findings are indicative of greater renal stress, as spontaneous blood and urine samples were obtained before and after exercise, whereas 24 hr samples are necessary to evaluate creatinine clearance.

Analysis of the available literature indicates that acute or chronic creatine supplementation (up to 10 weeks) does not appear to increase renal stress, as evaluated by various urine and serum markers, in healthy individuals. Additionally, no adverse effects of low-dose (1.5 g), long-term (1-5 years) creatine supplementation on renal function have been reported in clinical trials. However, few studies have comprehensively evaluated the effects of creatine on renal function, necessitating additional research before definitive conclusions can be offered.

Vandenberghe and coworkers (1997a) evaluated the effects of acute (20 g/day for 4 days) and chronic (5 g/day for 66 days) creatine supplementation on serum and urine markers of renal stress. Twenty-four-hour urine samples were collected prior to and following 1 and 3 days of creatine loading (20 g/day) and at 5 weeks and 10 weeks of lower-dose intake (5 g/day). Results revealed that during the acute loading phase, urinary creatine levels increased from 0.035 to 6.9 and 10.9 g/24 hr while urine creatinine levels increased from 1.19 to 1.44 and 1.56 g/24 hr from day 0 to days 1 and 3, respectively. After 10 weeks of low-dose supplementation (5 g/day), urine creatine (3.6 g/24 hr) and creatinine levels (1.56 g/24 hr) remained moderately elevated. Further, after cessation of creatine supplementation (20 g/day for 4 days and 5 g/day for 136 days), urine creatine and creatinine levels returned to baseline in four weeks. These findings indicate that the majority of excess creatine ingested during supplementation is excreted as creatine and that only a small amount of creatine is converted to creatinine. Moreover, there was no evidence that short- or long-term creatine supplementation (up to 10 weeks) impaired renal function.

Kreider and colleagues (1999b) reported initial findings from an open-label study addressing the long-term medical safety of creatine supplementation among athletes. In this study, 34 National Collegiate Athletic Association (NCAA) Division IA football players ingested three doses per day of Phosphagen HP™ containing 15.75 g/day of creatine for 5 days; they then ingested 5.25 g/day of creatine for 20 days prior to reporting to fall football camp. Nineteen subjects were provided a low-calorie carbohydrate-protein supplement containing no creatine. Training during phase I consisted of 4 to 5 days per week (70 min per workout) of resistance training indoors and sprint/agility conditioning outdoors. Training during phase II involved practice two to three times per day for 1.5 to 3.5 hr (207 min/day, 6 days per week) during 14 days of preseason football camp. During phase II, subjects in the creatine group were administered Phosphagain 2® containing 8.3 g/day of creatine. Prior to and following each phase of training, subjects donated fasting blood and 24 hr urine samples. Serum and urinary creatine and creatinine were determined, with renal function assessed by creatinine clearance. Results revealed no significant differences between creatine and non-creatine users in urinary creatinine excretion or creatinine clearance. These findings suggest that creatine supplementation during 25 days of preseason conditioning training and 14 days of fall two/three-a-day football camp does not affect markers of renal stress in well-trained athletes.

Finally, two recent studies attempted to determine whether long-term creatine users demonstrated evidence of increased renal stress in comparison to non-users. Poortmans and Francaux (1999) assessed kidney function in athletes who were chronic creatine consumers (10 months to 5 years) and controls. Subjects were assessed for plasma and urinary excretion rates of creatinine, urea, and albumin. Results revealed no significant differences between creatine users and non-users in these markers of kidney function indicating that glomular filtration rate, tubular reabsorption rate, and glomular membrane permeability were normal for both groups. In a similar study, Kreider et al. (1999c) evaluated creatinine clearance rates in 79 Division IA college football players (19.6 yrs, 72.5 in, 101.2 kg). The relationship between the subjects' history of taking creatine and markers of renal function was analyzed by Pearson Product-Moment correlation analysis. In addition, subjects were classified as non-users (n= 22), former users (n=40) and current creatine users (n = 17) to determine whether significant differences were observed in renal responses. Reported creatine use was 0.0, 5, and 1.3 months for the non-users, former users, and current users, respectively, with a range of 0 to 36 months of supplementation. Correlation analysis revealed that creatine use history was not correlated to urine creatinine levels or creatinine clearance. Moreover, no differences were observed among groups in urinary creatinine levels and creatinine clearance and all values were within normal ranges for athletes. The authors concluded that current and former creatine use does not significantly affect renal responses in healthy athletes.

In summary, analysis of available literature indicates that acute and chronic (up to 5 years) creatine supplementation does not appear to increase renal stress in healthy individuals. Additionally, no adverse effects of low-dose, long-term creatine supplementation (1.5 g/day for 1 to 5 years) on renal function have been reported in clinical trials (Sipilä et al. 1981; Vannas-Sulonen et al. 1985). It should be noted, however, that few studies have comprehensively evaluated the effects of creatine on renal function. Consequently, additional research using more precise methods of assessing renal function (e.g., insulin clearance) is warranted before definitive conclusions can be drawn.

Muscle and Liver Enzymes

Elevations in muscle and liver enzymes are often used as indicators of muscle, heart, and liver stress. Pathologically, these enzymes may be markedly elevated in response to degenerative muscle disease, myocardial infarction, and/or liver disease. Intense exercise also increases muscle and liver enzyme efflux, and muscle enzyme efflux is often used as an indicator of exercise intensity and training stress.

Several studies have evaluated the effects of creatine supplementation on muscle and liver enzyme efflux in sedentary and physically active subjects. Most studies show that creatine supplementation has no effect on creatine kinase (CK), lactate dehydrogenase (LDH), aspartate amino transferase (AST), alanine amino transferase (ALT), and gamma-glutamyl transaminase levels (Almada et al. 1996; Engelhardt et al. 1998; Kurosawa et al. 1997, 1998b; Mihic et al. 1998; Ransom et al. 1999; Sipilä et al. 1981).

Almada et al. (1996) reported that although no overall differences were observed when male and female values were analyzed together, physically active middle-aged men experienced mild elevations in CK (about 50%) during 8 weeks of creatine supplementation (20 g/day for 5 days and 10 g/day for 51 days), with no differences observed in women. These values returned to normal after 4-week cessation of creatine supplementation. Similar findings were reported by Kreider et al. (1998b), who found that football players ingesting creatine (15.75 g/day for 28 days) during intense resistance/agility training experienced significantly greater increases in CK (159% vs. 70%), LDH (24% vs. 11%), and ALT (17% vs. –7.3%) levels in comparison to the placebo group. The values observed, however, were well within normal ranges observed for athletes. The researchers suggested that the elevations in CK observed may reflect a greater concentration or activity of CK, an ability to maintain greater training volume, or both. More recent findings from the initial phases of an open-label long-term creatine safety study from this same research group, however, do not support their prior findings. In this regard, although CK levels were elevated during training in both groups, no significant differences were observed between creatine users and nonusers in serum CK, LDH, AST, or ALT levels during 25 days of preseason resistance/sprint training and during 14 days of fall two/three-a-day football camp (Ransom et al. 1999).

Research findings suggest that creatine supplementation does not affect muscle and liver enzyme efflux, elevations of which may be indicators of muscle, heart, or liver stress. However, some studies have shown increased serum levels of CK following creatine supplementation, which may possibly reflect an increased ability of subjects to train more intensely after supplementation. Nevertheless, additional research should be conducted to evaluate the effects of creatine on serum enzyme efflux in trained and nontrained populations.

Interestingly, in several of the studies in which creatine was administered to subjects not undergoing intense training, creatine supplementation did not significantly affect serum muscle enzyme efflux (Engelhardt et al. 1998; Kurosawa et al. 1998b; Mihic et al. 1998; Sipilä et al. 1981). These findings suggest that creatine supplementation does not affect muscle and liver enzyme efflux and that the increase in muscle and liver enzyme efflux previously reported may simply be a result of subjects training harder in response to creatine supplementation. However, two of these studies used relatively small doses of creatine daily, so additional research should be conducted to evaluate the effects of creatine on serum enzyme efflux in trained and nontrained populations.

Blood Volume and Electrolytes

Since muscle creatine uptake is sodium dependent and there have been some anecdotal reports that creatine may promote dehydration, muscle cramping, or both (see discussion later in this chapter), there has been recent interest in determining whether creatine supplementation affects blood volume or electrolyte status. Although data are limited, available studies indicate that short- and/or long-term creatine supplementation does not affect blood volume or serum electrolyte status (Harris et al. 1992; Kreider et al. 1998c; Ööpik et al. 1998; Rasmussen et al. 1999; Sipilä et al. 1981; Vannas-Sulonen et al. 1985).

For example, Harris et al. (1992) reported that ingesting 20-30 g/day of creatine for up to 10 days, or 30 g/day on alternating days for 21 days, did not affect blood profiles. Kreider et al. (1998c) reported that 28 days of creatine supplementation (15.75 g/day) during off-season college football resistance/agility training did not significantly affect fasting hematocrit, hemoglobin, sodium, chloride, potassium, calcium, or phosphorus levels. Ööpik and colleagues (1998) reported that creatine supplementation (20 g/day) during 5 days of rapid weight loss (3-4.3%) in well-trained karate athletes did not significantly affect fasting or postexercise hematocrit and plasma volume. Rasmussen and colleagues (1999) reported that creatine supplementation during preseason college football conditioning (15.75 g/day for 5 days and 5.25 g/day for 20 days) and fall two/three-a-day football camp (8.3 g/day for 14 days) conducted in a hot and humid environment (33.7°C, 79% relative humidity [RH]) did not significantly affect fasting serum sodium, chloride, potassium, calcium, phosphorus, plasma volume, or blood volume in comparison to the corresponding values in athletes not ingesting creatine. Finally, no significant effects of long-term, low-dose creatine supplementation (1.5 g/day for 1 to 5 years) on electrolyte status or blood volume were reported by Sipilä and colleagues (1981) or Vannas-Sulonen and coworkers (1985). Collectively, these studies indicate that creatine supplementation does not appear to affect electrolyte status or blood volume.

Muscle creatine uptake is sodium dependent, so creatine supplementation theoretically may influence electrolyte status, blood volume, or both. However, available studies indicate that short-term or long-term creatine supplementation does not affect serum electrolyte status or blood volume.

Blood Pressure

Since creatine supplementation has been associated with weight gain, some concern has been raised regarding whether creatine supplementation may adversely affect blood pressure. However, although limited, studies evaluating the effects of short-term and long-term creatine supplementation on blood pressure have shown no effect despite significant increases in total body weight, lean body mass, or both (Mihic et al. 1998; Peeters et al. 1998; Sipilä et al. 1981; Vannas-Sulonen et al. 1985).

Lipid Profiles

It has been reported that creatine supplementation positively affects lipid profiles in middle-aged male and female hypertriglyceremic patients (Earnest et al. 1996a) and trained male athletes (Kreider et al. 1998b; Melton et al. 1999). In this regard, Earnest et al. (1996a) reported that 56 days of creatine supplementation resulted in significant decreases in total cholesterol (–5% and –6% at day 28 and 56, respectively) and triglycerides (–23% and –22% at day 28 and 56, respectively) in mildly hypertriglyceremic subjects. A similar response was observed with very low density lipoproteins (VLDL). In addition, Kreider and coworkers (1998b) reported that 28 days of creatine supplementation during training increased high-density lipoproteins (HDL) by 13% while decreasing VLDL (–13%) and the ratio of total cholesterol to HDL (–7%). Finally, Melton and colleagues (1999) reported that college football players ingesting creatine-containing supplements during two phases of preseason college football training showed significant decreases in total cholesterol (creatine –10% vs. control –2%) and low-density lipoprotein levels (creatine –12% vs. control 1%) after 42 days of supplementation (15.75 g/day for 5 days, 5.25 g/day for 20 days, and 8.3 g/day for 17 days) in comparison to controls. These findings suggest that creatine supplementation may possess some health benefit by improving blood lipid profiles. However, creatine supplementation (25g/day for 7 days and 5 g/day for 77 days) has also been shown to have no effect on serum profiles (Lawson et al. 1998). Possible differences in creatine dosage and/or type of training may account for these equivocal findings. Additional research is merited.

Some findings suggest that creatine supplementation may offer some health benefit by improving blood lipid profiles, but more research is needed to confirm these preliminary findings.

Medical Uses of Creatine and Phosphocreatine

Although the recent focus of creatine supplementation has been on determining the potential ergogenic value, a significant body of research has evaluated various medical uses of creatine and PCr. The following overview describes some of the potential therapeutic uses of creatine and PCr supplementation and/or administration in various patient populations.

Creatine Synthesis Deficiencies

As mentioned in chapter 2, creatine is stored in skeletal muscle and brain. The availability of creatine and PCr is essential to maintain normal metabolic and neurological function. Some children are born with an inefficiency in synthesizing creatine or an inability to synthesize it (Arias-Mendosa et al. 1998). The net effect is that total body and brain concentrations of creatine and PCr are significantly decreased, resulting in impaired motor and mental function. Since oral creatine supplements became available, creatine supplementation (4 to 8 g/day for up to 25 months) has been used to treat infants with inborn errors in creatine synthesis (Stöckler and Hanefeld 1997; Stöckler et al. 1994, 1996a, 1996b). Results from these studies show that oral creatine supplementation serves to normalize total body and brain creatine and PCr stores. Moreover, the infants treated with oral creatine supplementation experienced more normal mental and physical development, with no apparent side effects reported.

Gyrate Atrophy

Gyrate atrophy of the choroid and retina is a relatively rare autosomal-recessive tapetoretinal disease that is associated with night blindness, atrophy of the fundi, reduction of visual fields, myopia, and cataracts (Sipilä et al. 1981). This condition typically results in blindness by early middle age (30 to 40 yr). The condition is also associated with a gradual atrophy of type II muscle fiber and an increase in tubular aggregates from the affected fibers. This atrophy has been attributed to an hyperornithinemia-induced inhibition of creatine synthesis. The result is that patients with gyrate atrophy have markedly reduced tissue concentrations of creatine and PCr.

On the basis of these observations, oral creatine supplementation (1.5 g/day for 1 to 5 years) has been used as a therapeutic treatment for gyrate atrophy patients (Sipilä et al. 1981; Vannas-Sulonen et al. 1985). Results of these studies revealed that creatine supplementation (1.5 g/day for 1 year) served to reduce the number of affected fibers by about 10% as well as to decrease the number and frequency of tubular aggregates. This was accompanied by a delay in progression of visual impairment. No side effects were reported. In the 5-year follow-up analysis, abnormalities in skeletal muscle decreased or rapidly disappeared with creatine supplementation. Although progression of gyrate atrophy occurred, there appeared to be less progression in patients with advanced stages of the disease. Again, no significant side effects were noted. These findings suggest that low-dose creatine supplementation may provide therapeutic value to gyrate atrophy patients with hyperornithine-induced creatine synthesis deficiencies.

Heart Disease

An extensive amount of research has been conducted on the potential medical benefits of intravenous PCr administration and oral creatine supplementation in patients with heart disease. A detailed analysis of the clinical applications of PCr and creatine can be found in the recent book by Conway and Clark (1996a). Basically, intravenous PCr administration has been reported to improve myocardial metabolism and reduce the incidence of ventricular fibrillation in ischemic heart patients (Andrews et al. 1998; Constantin-Teodosiu et al. 1995; Conway et al. 1996a; Ferraro et al. 1996; Horn et al. 1998; Gordon et al. 1995; Pauletto and Strumia 1996; Saks 1996; Saks et al. 1996; Schaufelberger and Swedberg 1998). The reason is that PCr appears to enhance the viability of the ischemic cell membrane, thereby minimizing cell injury during ischemia. Consequently, intravenous administration of PCr has been used effectively as a cardioprotective therapy in heart patients (Saks et al. 1996).

There has also been interest in determining the effects of oral creatine supplementation on heart function and exercise capacity in patients with chronic heart failure. The rationale is that creatine supplementation may serve to enhance myocardial and/or skeletal muscle metabolic efficiency. Gordon and associates (1995) reported that creatine supplementation (20 g/day for 10 days) did not improve ejection fraction in heart failure patients who had an ejection fraction less than 40%. However, creatine supplementation significantly increased one-legged knee extension exercise performance (21%), peak torque (5%), and cycle ergometry performance (10%) in these patients.

More recently, Andrews and coworkers (1998) investigated the effects of oral creatine supplementation (20 g/day for 5 days) on skeletal muscle metabolism in patients with congestive heart failure. Subjects performed 5 sec isometric handgrip contractions, followed by 5 sec of resting recovery, for 5 min at 25%, 50%, and 75% of maximal voluntary contraction. The researchers found that isometric force was increased following creatine supplementation. Additionally, forearm ammonia and lactate concentrations were decreased in the creatine group. The investigators concluded that creatine supplementation in chronic heart failure patients improves skeletal muscle endurance and attenuates the abnormal skeletal muscle metabolic response to exercise.

Collectively, these studies suggest that intravenous PCr administration may provide cardioprotective benefit to patients with ischemic heart disease. Further, they indicate that oral creatine supplementation may enhance exercise tolerance in patients with chronic congestive heart failure. Additional research should be conducted to evaluate these potential therapeutic benefits of PCr and creatine administration.

Neuromuscular Disease

Creatine deficiencies have been reported in a variety of neuromuscular diseases (Kent-Braun et al. 1994; Khanna and Madan, 1978; Matthews et al. 1998; Pulido et al. 1998; Sipilä et al. 1981; Tarnopolsky et al. 1997; Tarnopolsky and Martin 1999; Vannas-Sulonen et al. 1985; Whittinham and Lipton 1991; Wyss et al. 1998). Consequently there has been recent interest in determining whether creatine supplementation may provide therapeutic benefit to patients with mitochondrial cytopathies, Huntington's disease, multiple sclerosis, and muscle dystrophies.

Although this area of creatine research is in its infancy, there are several published reports which suggest that creatine supplementation may provide therapeutic benefit for patients with neuromuscular disease. In this regard, Tarnopolsky and colleagues (1997) reported that creatine supplementation (5 g/day for 14 days followed by 2 g/day for 7 days) significantly increased anaerobic and high-intensity aerobic exercise capacity in patients with mitochondrial cytopathy (a neuromuscular disease associated with poor exercise capacity). Additionally, Tarnopolsky and Martin (1999) reported that creatine supplementation (10 g/day for 5 days to 5 g/day for 5 days) increased body weight, handgrip, dorsiflexion, and knee extension strength in patients with neuromuscular disease. Moreover, Pulido et al. (1998) reported that creatine treatment in mice with abnormally elevated cytosolic calcium concentrations associated with Duchenne muscular dystrophy served to normalize these calcium concentrations by stimulating sarcoplasmic reticulum calcium APTase activity. These findings suggest that creatine supplementation may be useful for treatment of Duchenne muscular dystrophy. Consequently, there appears to be some promising therapeutic benefit of creatine supplementation in patients with neuromuscular disease.

Orthopedic Rehabilitation

Creatine supplementation has been shown to promote muscle fiber hypertrophy and greater gains in strength during resistance training (see chapters 5 and 8).

Consequently, there has been recent interest in determining whether creatine supplementation before and/or after orthopedic injury or surgery may reduce atrophy, facilitate faster recovery during rehabilitation, or both. Although research addressing this hypothesis is in its infancy, there are at least two reports that provide support. First, Satolli and Marchesi (1989) reported that creatine phosphate administration increased muscle girth of the thigh after knee surgery. In addition, in a study by Pirola et al. (1991), older patients (over 60 years) who experienced muscle atrophy after fracture of the femur showed a 1.9-fold greater increase in echotomography-determined thigh and leg muscle mass when receiving intramuscular PCr supplementation (500 mg/day for 20 days) in conjunction with physical therapy, as compared to subjects not receiving creatine phosphate. We are also aware that research is currently under way to evaluate the effects of oral creatine supplementation on atrophy rates and rehabilitation outcomes following injury or leg immobilization. Additional research should address this potential therapeutic role of PCr and creatine supplementation.

Creatine supplementation has been used therapeutically for the treatment of various medical disorders, including creatine synthesis deficiencies, gyrate atrophy, heart disease, neuromuscular disease, and orthopedic rehabilitation.

Tumor Growth Inhibition

Preliminary research in animals suggests that dietary availability of creatine may inhibit growth rate of certain tumors. In this regard, Miller et al. (1993) evaluated the effects on mice fed with diets containing 1% cyclocreatine or 1, 2, 5, or 10% creatine. The investigators evaluated the growth rates of rat mammary tumors, sarcoma in male rats, and tumors from two forms of human neuroblastoma cell lines injected subcutaneously in mice. Results revealed that dietary creatine availability may delay the appearance of tumors in rats and mice. However, additional research with animals and humans is necessary to further explore this potential medical benefit.

Anecdotally Reported Side Effects

Weight gain is the only side effect reported from clinical research studies involving dosages ranging from 35 g/day for 3 days to 1.5 g/day for 5 years in diseased populations, untrained subjects, and athletes (Balsom et al. 1994; Kreider 1998a; Plisk and Kreider 1999; Williams and Branch 1998). However, a number of undocumented anecdotal reports of possible side effects of creatine supplementation have appeared in lay publications and in the media (Armour 1998; Gola 1998; Hellmich 1998a, 1998b; Mihoces 1998; O'Donnell and Mihoces 1998; Strauss and Mihoces 1998). In addition, 20 possible adverse events or side effects of ingesting creatine-containing supplements (with or without other supplements or nutrients) were listed in the report of the Food and Drug Administration (FDA) Special Nutritionals Adverse Event Monitoring System of May 14, 1998. This report is available online at: **http://vm.cfsan.fda.gov/~dms/aems.html**.

Heightened attention developed with reported suspicions that one of three wrestlers who died suddenly in the winter of 1997 of heat exhaustion, dehydration, and/or heart failure after intense workouts in a hot environment, in an attempt to lose weight rapidly, may have used creatine (Associated Press 1997a, 1997b, 1998d). On the basis of these suspicions, it was reported that the FDA was going to investigate whether or not creatine supplementation may have been a contributing factor in these deaths (Associated Press 1997b).

Since then, hundreds of newspaper, magazine, and Internet articles have been written about the safety of creatine supplementation. Additionally, several national television shows in the United States aired feature stories regarding creatine supplementation. In many of these stories, reporters asked athletes, trainers, coaches, scientists, or physicians to offer opinions regarding creatine use among athletes. Unfortunately, many of these anecdotal reports presented inaccurate information about the safety and efficacy of creatine supplementation. For example, although no side effects were reported in any scientific study, it was stated in numerous articles that creatine supplementation causes muscle cramping, muscle tears, dehydration, diarrhea, or a combination of these (Gola 1998; Hellmich 1998b; Strauss and Mihoces 1998; Strauss 1998; *USA Today* Editorial 1998). Additionally, in a front-page story in *USA Today* it was reported that the FDA had issued a warning on the use of creatine (O'Donnell and Mihoces 1998). The FDA, however, issued a statement indicating that there was no such warning specifically about creatine and that the FDA was not investigating creatine at all. Additionally, the FDA issued a report containing the conclusion that creatine had been ruled out as a primary factor in the death of these wrestlers (Associated Press 1998a).

In large part as a result of these reports, numerous athletic governing bodies and professional organizations have begun to evaluate their supplementation policies. Some schools and organizations have banned creatine administration to athletes. Others have issued position statements warning their athletes of side effects of creatine supplementation (Strauss 1998). Still others have implemented supervised administration policies (Plisk and Kreider 1999). More recently, the ethics of athletes who take "drugs" like creatine have been questioned (Associated Press 1998b, 1998c; Dixon 1998). Chapter 10 presents a discussion of some of the legal and ethical issues related to creatine supplementation.

It should be noted that the concerns about creatine supplementation that have been described in the popular media or reported to the FDA's Special Nutritionals Adverse Event Monitoring System (SN/AEMS) emanate from anecdotal reports and may be unrelated to creatine supplementation. In fact, the FDA suggests the following when one is interpreting adverse reactions or side effects reported to the SN/AEMS system:

> "There is no certainty that a reported adverse event can be attributed to a particular product or ingredient. The available information may not be complete enough to make this determination.
>
> Reporting of an adverse event may be affected by many factors, including length of time a product or ingredient has been marketed or publicity."

In the case of creatine, no evidence from any well-controlled clinical study indicates that creatine supplementation causes any of the side effects that have been reported anecdotally. Some anecdotal evidence, as derived from a recent survey conducted by the National Strength and Conditioning Association (NSCA), actually indicates no serious problems with creatine supplementation. The majority of the coaches and trainers surveyed, all NSCA members, indicated that the use of creatine is a safe way to increase the intensity of training for serious athletes, including high school athletes (Associated Press 1998e). In our opinion, comments regarding the effects or side effects of creatine should be based on scientific evidence, not speculation. In this regard, Bolotte (1998) indicated that although many scientific studies have addressed the ergogenic effects of creatine supplementation and no deleterious effects have been proven as of yet, many physicians who work with athletes are advising caution. Thus, one must consider that although there are few reported side effects from these scientific publications, few long-term studies on creatine supplementation have been conducted. It is possible that creatine abuse (i.e., taking excessive amounts of creatine), poor quality of creatine supplements, and/or interactions with other factors such as consuming multiple dietary supplements may account for some of these anecdotal observations (Plisk and Kreider 1999). It is also possible that adverse reactions to creatine supplementation may occur in some people under conditions that have yet to be clinically investigated. Consequently, analysis of the scientific validity of anecdotally reported side effects is warranted.

Gastrointestinal Distress

There have been some anecdotal reports that creatine supplementation may cause gastrointestinal (GI) distress (i.e., stomach upset, gas, diarrhea, etc.). The theory suggests that although creatine is absorbed intact from the gut (see chapter 2), there may be an upper limit to intestinal absorption of creatine. If this is so, then the excess creatine ingested may serve to cause gas and loose stools and/or diarrhea.

Analysis of the available scientific literature, however, does not support this view, in that no study has shown creatine supplementation to have caused significant GI distress when taken at the recommended doses (about 5 to 8 g per serving up to 35 g/day). Reports of GI distress from creatine studies have been isolated and rare, and not significant enough to cause removal of subjects from the protocols. Moreover, in an analysis of five of their creatine studies, Kreider and associates (1998c) recently found that reports of GI distress in subjects administered creatine-containing supplements were isolated and were fewer than for subjects taking placebo supplements. However, it is also possible that individuals consuming doses of creatine that have not been studied (i.e., > 10 g per serving and/or > 35 g/day) might experience GI distress. Additionally, it is possible that other ingredients in some of the creatine-containing supplements may cause GI distress in some people. Nevertheless, given the widespread use of creatine, it does not appear that creatine causes an amount of GI distress sufficient to diminish its popularity among athletes.

Muscle Cramping and Dehydration

Probably the most commonly reported anecdotal side effect from creatine supplementation is a greater incidence of dehydration, muscle cramps, or heat intolerance in athletes who train hard in hot and humid environments (Strauss 1998). It is possible that since creatine may allow an athlete to train more intensely, this may predispose one to dehydration and/or heat injury. However, the prevalent theory

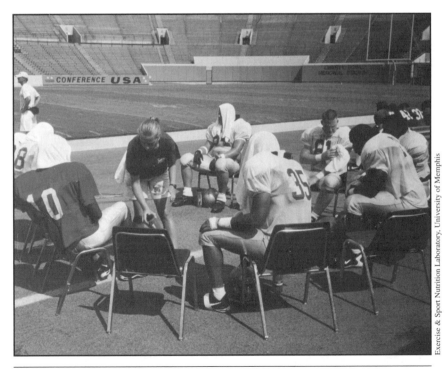

Exercise & Sport Nutrition Laboratory, University of Memphis

Figure 9.1   Division IA football players attempting to tolerate the heat and humidity during a fall football camp scrimmage.

suggests that water retention during the early phases of creatine supplementation may underlie these anecdotal reports (Clark 1997). Theoretically it is conceivable that an increase in intracellular water, as noted in chapter 8, could disturb the normal intracellular electrolyte balance, inducing muscle cramps. However, creatine supplementation does not appear to lead to dehydration, but actually a greater body water content.

Based on these anecdotal reports, some athletic organizations have published position statements on creatine supplementation for their athletes. The following are some excerpts from such a statement provided by the Tampa Bay Buccaneers of the National Football League, published in *USA Today* (Strauss 1998).

"Creatine supplementation may cause an electrolyte imbalance, specifically reversing the normal calcium:phosphorus ratio, interfering with the muscle's contraction/relaxation mechanisms, possibly causing cramping.

This electrolyte imbalance may also predispose athletes to dehydration and heat-related illness. Increased fluid retention within the muscle cells reduces blood plasma volume, which may adversely affect one's ability to perform and dissipate heat."

It should be noted, however, that no scientific data support these statements. No study has reported that creatine supplementation causes severe cramping or dehydration, significantly alters electrolyte status, affects the calcium:phosphorus ratio, or decreases plasma volume or blood volume. This is true even though many of these studies have evaluated highly trained athletes undergoing intense exercise in hot and humid environments (see the previous section on blood volume and electrolytes).

Anecdotal reports have linked creatine supplementation to various health problems, including GI distress, muscle cramping, dehydration, and muscle injury. Although there appear to be no clinical data to support these anecdotal reports, and actually some data to refute them, well-controlled research is needed to evaluate these anecdotally reported effects.

Several recent studies also directly refute these anecdotal reports. No study that has evaluated the effects of acute or chronic creatine supplementation on total body water has shown that creatine promotes dehydration (Hultman et al. 1996; Kreider et al. 1996a, 1998b; Podewils 1998; Ziegenfuss et al. 1998b). In fact, creatine supplementation has been reported to promote a mild fluid retention; in most cases the gain in total body water was proportional to weight gains. Moreover, Ööpik and associates (1998) reported that creatine supplementation (20 g/day for 5 days) during a period in which athletes were attempting to rapidly reduce body weight (3-4.3%) mitigated the ability of the athletes to lose weight. These findings indicate that creatine may help prevent dehydration rather than promote dehydration. The researchers suggested that since creatine supplementation has been found to increase body weight and body water, it may be more difficult for athletes to lose weight rapidly when taking creatine. Thus, it is important that athletes involved in weight-control sports should be aware that creatine supplementation may impede their ability to make weight, and they need to be educated regarding inappropriate weight-loss techniques so that they do not attempt to employ inappropriate and potentially dangerous weight-loss methods to counteract this effect.

In an attempt to evaluate retrospectively whether creatine supplementation was associated with cramping, Kreider and coworkers (1998c) examined poststudy questionnaires from subjects participating in five previous creatine studies. During these studies, athletes were involved in weight training (28 days, ~8 hr per week), swim training (9 days, ~21 hr per week), off-season football resistance/agility training (28 to 35 days, ~8 hr per week), spring football practice (5 weeks, ~20 hr per week), and endurance training (14 days, ~12 to 20 hr per week of cycling, running, or both). During the studies, subjects ingested supplements containing 15 to 25 g/day of creatine or placebos in a double-blind and randomized manner. After the studies, subjects completed poststudy questionnaires in a double-blind manner. Subjects were asked to report positive and negative aspects of the supplements they took as well as any side effects. Examination of results revealed no reports of cramping in creatine or non-creatine users.

Authors of two recent studies have attempted to directly evaluate the effects of creatine supplementation on hydration status and cramping during exercising in the heat. Podewils (1998), in a double-blind and randomized manner, assigned 20 males to a creatine group (20 g/day for 5 days and 10 g/day thereafter) or a placebo group for 28 days. Total body weight and bioelectrical impedance-determined total body water were ascertained at weekly intervals. In addition, subjects exercised at 60% of $\dot{V}O_{2max}$ for 60 min in an environmental chamber (37 °C, 25% RH) before and after supplementation. Results revealed that creatine supplementation increased total body weight by 1.9 kg and total body water by 2.2 L. The gain in total body weight was not significantly greater than that in controls, whereas the increase in total body water was significantly greater. In addition, core temperature during exercise tended to interact between groups (p = 0.052), with core temperature decreasing in the creatine group and increasing in the control group. The researcher hypothesized that the creatine-enhanced fluid retention may have served to attenuate increases in core temperature during exercise in the heat. No incidents of cramping were reported. These findings indicate that creatine supplementation does not negatively affect core temperature, promote dehydration, or cause cramping when a person is performing moderate-intensity exercise in the heat, and may even be protective against heat stress.

Finally, preliminary reports from the initial phases of a long-term open-label creatine safety study do not support contentions that creatine supplementation during training in a hot and humid environment promotes dehydration or increases the incidence of cramping (Rasmussen et al. 1999; Kreider et al. 1999a; Hunt et al. 1999). In this regard, Division IA college football players were monitored during two phases of preseason training. During precamp training, 77 athletes underwent

4 to 5 days per week (mean = 70 min per workout) of resistance training indoors (mean = 28 °C, 79% RH) and sprint/agility conditioning outdoors (mean = 32 °C, 84% RH). During fall football camp, 99 athletes practiced two to three times per day (mean = 207 min/day, 6 days per week) in environmental conditions averaging 33.7°C and 79% RH. During precamp training, 34 of 77 athletes (44%) ingested three servings per day of Phosphagen HP™ containing 15.75 g/day of creatine for five days and then ingested one serving per day (5.25 g/day of creatine) for 20 days. During the 14-day camp, 34 of 99 subjects (35%) ingested one serving per day of Phosphagain 2® containing 8.3 g of creatine. The remaining subjects were provided a low-calorie carbohydrate-protein supplement with no creatine. Cramping and heat injuries treated by the athletic training staff were recorded. Results revealed that the incidence of cramping for the creatine users was 0 of 1 (0%) during precamp training and 17 of 49 (35%) during camp. The incidence of heat illness/dehydration episodes was 0 of 0 (0%) during precamp training and 3 of 8 (38%) during camp. The observed incidence of cramping and dehydration episodes was generally proportional to or lower than the creatine use rate among players during precamp conditioning (44%) and fall camp (35%). In addition, no significant differences were observed between creatine users (n = 34) and non-users (n = 19) in 24 hr urine volume, urine specific gravity, or electrolyte status (Rasmussen et al. 1999). These findings indicate that creatine supplementation (5.25 to 15.75 g/day) during preseason college football training in hot and humid environmental conditions does not promote dehydration or increase the incidence of cramping in comparison to what occurs in non-users.

In summary, although anecdotal reports suggest that creatine supplementation during intense training may promote dehydration and increase the incidence of muscle cramping, available scientific evidence does not support these contentions. Nevertheless, additional research should be performed to evaluate the validity of these anecdotal reports.

Muscle Injury

There have also been some anecdotal reports that creatine supplementation may promote a greater incidence of muscle strains or pulls (Gola 1998; Hellmich 1998b; Strauss 1998). The theory is that since creatine supplementation may promote relatively rapid gains in strength and body mass, additional stress may be placed on bone, joints, and ligaments, leading to injury. These reports have primarily emanated from athletic trainers' observations of what they perceive to be an increased incidence of certain types of injury (e.g., hamstring pulls). Currently, available studies have not shown an increased incidence rate of injuries in response to creatine supplementation, even though many of these studies evaluated highly trained athletes during periods of heavy training. Further, no study has documented a greater rate of injury during training in creatine users than in non-users.

Several recent groups have attempted to evaluate the incidence of injury among athletes taking creatine. Kreider et al. (1998c) state that no subjects from five of their previous studies reported a creatine-related musculoskeletal injury in response to creatine supplementation. Additionally, preliminary findings from a long-term open-label creatine safety study indicate that creatine supplementation during two phases of preseason college football training decreased the incidence of injury when adjusted for the use rate of creatine among players (Kreider et al. 1999a; Hunt et al. 1999). In this regard, with use of the methods described earlier, the incidence of injuries treated by the athletic training staff was monitored during 25 days of precamp resistance/sprint conditioning and during 14 days of fall two/three-a-day football camp. Results revealed that the incidence (creatine/non-creatine, percentage of injuries in creatine users) of precamp muscle pulls/strains (0/3, 0%), noncontact joint injuries (0/1, 0%), and total treated injuries (1/8, 13%) was lower than the creatine use rate among players during precamp conditioning (44%). During fall football camp, the incidence of muscle pulls/strains (1/7, 14%), noncontact joint injuries (7/22, 32%), contact injuries (4/11, 36%), and illness (1/10, 10%), as well as the number of missed practices due to injury (26/70, 38%) and total injuries/missed practices (64/188, 34%), was generally proportional to or lower than the creatine use rate among players during fall camp (35%). Moreover, when data were statistically normalized for use rate among athletes, the creatine users had a significantly lower observed injury/illness rate in comparison to their use rate whereas non-users showed an inverse relationship. These findings indicate that creatine supplementation (5.25 to 15.75 g/day) does not increase the incidence of injury during preseason college football training.

In summary, although many groups of researchers have evaluated athletes during intense training, there is no current evidence that creatine supplementation promotes muscle injury. Nevertheless, the validity of anecdotal reports should be evaluated in additional research.

Long-Term Safety

A significant amount of concern has been expressed regarding unknown long-term side effects of creatine supplementation. This concern has been perpetuated primarily in lay articles and in the media. In response, several athletic governing boards (e.g., NCAA, United States Olympic Committee, etc.) have been reported to be considering legislation to restrict creatine administration to their athletes because of legal or ethical issues, or both (see chapter 10). Although long-term safety data are limited, particularly in athletes, the literature contains reports of several long-term trials indicating that creatine supplementation is safe for a variety of populations.

Vannas-Sulonen and colleagues (1985) reported no adverse side effects of low-dose creatine supplementation (1.5 g/day for 5 years) in gyrate atrophy patients. According to Dr. Sipilä, a member of this research group, many of the patients evaluated in these reports have continued to take creatine (1.5 to 3 g/day) with no significant medical complications observed over the 17-year supplementation period (personal commmunication). Further, creatine supplementation (4 to 8 g/day for up to 25 months) has been used to treat infants with creatine synthesis deficiencies with no side effects reported (Stöckler and Hanefeld 1997; Stöckler et al. 1994, 1996a, 1996b). It is interesting to note that this dosage would be equivalent to an adult dosage of 0.5 to 1.5 g/kg/day (35 to 105 g/day for a 70 kg person). Extensive research has also been conducted on the cardioprotective effects of PCr administration and oral creatine supplementation in chronic heart failure patients (Saks et al. 1996). Collectively, these long-term data indicate that creatine supplementation is safe.

Health professionals have expressed concern regarding unknown long-term side effects of creatine supplementation. Although no data are available to indicate adverse health effects associated with long-term creatine supplementation, at least when taken at dosages described in the literature, additional research is needed to evaluate its medical safety.

With regard to sport, athletes have been reported to be using creatine as a nutritional supplement since the mid-1960s (Gola 1998; Plisk and Kreider 1999). Yet, as of this writing, no significant medical complication has been directly linked to creatine supplementation. Additionally, preliminary data presented at the 1998 National Strength and Conditioning Association Annual Meeting (Larson et al. 1998) from Dr. Mike Stone's laboratory indicate that long-term creatine supplementation (up to 2 years) does not result in any abnormal clinical outcome in comparison to outcomes for controls. Similar findings were reported by Kreider et al. (1999c) in athletes taking creatine for up to 3 years and Poortmans and Francaux (1999) in athletes taking creatine for up to 5 years. Consequently, on the basis of available scientific research findings, creatine supplementation appears to pose no serious health risks when taken at dosages described in the literature. Nevertheless, additional research should be performed to evaluate the medical safety of long-term creatine supplementation among athletes.

Chapter Summary

Although creatine is a naturally occurring nutrient and athletes have been anecdotally reported to have been taking creatine supplements since the 1960s, its widespread use as a dietary supplement did not begin until the early to mid 1990s. Consequently, concern has been raised regarding its short- and long-term medical safety. Analysis of available literature indicates that the only side effect reported from creatine supplementation is weight gain. However, concerns have been raised regarding whether creatine supplementation results in long-term suppression of endogenous creatine synthesis, causes renal and liver damage, promotes dehydration, alters electrolyte status, increases blood pressure, causes GI upset, promotes severe muscle cramping, and/or promotes injury during training. Careful analysis of available literature indicates that although more research is needed, there is no scientific evidence to substantiate these concerns. Conversely, a number of studies report that creatine supplementation does not affect these concerns. Additionally, there is some evidence that creatine supplementation may favorably affect blood lipids as well as provide therapeutic benefit for patients with creatine synthesis deficiencies, gyrate atrophy, heart failure, neuromuscular diseases, and following orthopedic injury. Consequently, available studies indicate that creatine supplementation appears to pose no health risk in supplementation trials lasting up to 5-years in duration and may provide therapeutic benefit for certain patient populations.

Nevertheless some health professionals recommend additional research, particularly large randomized controlled studies evaluating both the short and long term effects of oral creatine supplements on the various organ systems in which creatine plays a metabolic role (Juhn and Tarnopolsky, 1998b). In the meantime, individuals, particularly those with pre-existing medical problems, should consult their physician before taking creatine, or for that matter, any dietary supplement.

10

CHAPTER

Legal and Ethical Issues Regarding Creatine Supplementation

From time immemorial, athletes have utilized a variety of methods in attempts to enhance performance (Wadler and Hainline 1989). For example, two social food drugs, alcohol and caffeine, were used for their ergogenic potential over 100 years ago (Williams 1974). During the past half-century, more potent drugs have become available and have been used increasingly by athletes. Strong stimulants, such as amphetamines, as well as anabolic/androgenic steroids were very popular in the 1960s and 1970s. After several ergogenic drug-related deaths, including one in the 1960 Rome Olympic Games, the International Olympic Committee (IOC) initiated its anti-drug, or doping, legislation. Currently, the IOC prohibits various classes of substances (stimulants, narcotics, anabolic agents, diuretics, and peptide and glycoprotein hormones and analogues), methods (blood doping and pharmacological, chemical, and physical manipulation), and classes of drugs subject to certain restrictions (alcohol, marijuana, local anesthetics, corticosteroids, and beta-blockers) (Cowan 1997).

Use of ergogenic drugs in elite sport competition has decreased dramatically in recent years following the advent of highly sophisticated and effective drug-detection techniques, primarily urinalysis via high-resolution mass spectrometry. Athletes have turned to effective substances that cannot be detected via current drug-testing procedures. Recombinant technology has led to mass production of two potential ergogenic hormones, recombinant human growth hormone (rHGH) and recombinant erythropoietin (rEPO). Research is currently under way to provide effective testing procedures for these agents in the year 2000 Olympic Games, but David A. Cowan (1997), a drug-testing expert from the United Kingdom, indicates

217

that a blood test will most likely be necessary. Currently, the International Cycling Federation uses a blood test for hematocrit determination, a possible marker for rEPO use, so it is possible that blood testing may be a viable means to counter the use of substances that may not be detected by current urinalysis testing.

Through advances in nutritional biotechnology, scientists have been able to synthesize or manufacture all known nutrients, and many of their metabolic by-products, essential to human physiology. Many of these nutrients or by-products are theorized to possess ergogenic potential when consumed in amounts well in excess of recommended daily intake. In this regard, some sports administrators believe that the line is getting thinner and thinner between proscribed and prescribed supplements and drugs (Associated Press 1993).

Legal Aspects

In the United States, the Dietary Health and Education Act (DSHEA) defines a dietary supplement as a food product, added to the total diet, that contains at least one of the following ingredients: a vitamin, mineral, herb or botanical, amino acid, metabolite, constituent, extract, or combination of any of these ingredients. It is important to note the stipulation in the DSHEA that dietary supplements cannot be represented as a conventional food or as a sole item of a meal or diet. As this definition indicates, dietary supplements may contain essential nutrients such as essential vitamins, minerals, and amino acids, but also other nonessential substances such as ginseng, ginkgo, yohimbe, ma huang, and other herbal products (Williams 1999).

Given the prohibition of drug use as a performance enhancer, many athletes resort to dietary supplements for potential ergogenic effects. Indeed, numerous dietary supplements are marketed to athletes and physically active individuals with the imputed effect of enhanced sport or exercise performance. For example, in a recent survey of only five magazines targeted to bodybuilding athletes, Grunewald and Bailey (1993) reported that more than 800 performance claims were made for 624 commercially available supplements ranging alphabetically from amino acids to yohimbine.

At the present time, no essential nutrient is classified as a drug, and all essential nutrients are considered to be legal for use in conjunction with athletic competition. Most other food substances and constituents sold as dietary supplements are also legal. However, several dietary supplements available in the United States are prohibited by the IOC. Numerous dietary supplements, such as ma huang or products marketed for weight loss, contain ephedra or ephedrine, an IOC-prohibited stimulant. Dehydroepiandrosterone and androstenedione, both natural precursors for testosterone, are marketed as dietary supplements, but their use is also prohibited by the IOC because they are substances that are related to anabolic steroids or that may mask their use.

Several reviewers (Greenhaff 1995; Maughan 1995) have indicated that creatine supplementation may be an effective ergogenic aid, and as noted in previous chapters of this monograph, the research data support these indications, at least for certain types of exercise performance. Indeed, Roger Harris, one of the principal creatine-supplementation investigators from Great Britain, has been quoted as saying, "Creatine could have an impact on world records. If you happen to be a world record-holder, one can only assume you will do better. It will be exciting to see this" (Associated Press 1993). Anecdotal information indicates that several Olympians used creatine supplementation for the 1992 Barcelona Olympic Games (Associated Press 1993).

Currently, creatine is considered a natural dietary constituent, and the IOC recently classified creatine as a food; its use as a supplement to enhance sport performance has not been prohibited by the IOC or other athletic governing organizations. Even if its use were prohibited, Greenhaff (1997a) noted that it is difficult to envisage how use could be detected without the availability of serial muscle biopsies over the course of several months. Urinary creatinine excretion is increased following creatine ingestion, but the daily variation in this measurement between and within individuals is large, and therefore measurements could offer only tentative indications of ingestion (Greenhaff 1997a).

Although noting that creatine is not on the IOC doping list, Ekblom (1996) indicated that many people regard creatine as a substance in the gray zone between doping and use of substances allowed to enhance performance. Given the fact that creatine supplementation is not prohibited by the IOC, its use by athletes is legal, but may raise some ethical issues.

Creatine is currently considered a natural dietary constituent and neither the IOC nor other athletic governing organizations have prohibited its use as a supplement to enhance sport performance. However, some contend that creatine falls in the gray zone between doping and use of substances allowed to enhance performance.

Ethical Aspects

Ethics may be defined in a variety of ways, one definition being the moral principles of a particular school of thought. In relation to sport, the ancient Greek belief that athletes should succeed through their own unaided effort is embraced by the IOC as the Olympic ideal. According to another definition, ethics is the rules of conduct recognized in particular associations. Within the IOC, certain associations establish specific rules for conduct within their sport, such as specific applications of the doping rule, to ensure that athletes adhere to the Olympic ideal and do not obtain an unfair advantage. In yet another definition, ethics consists of the moral principles by which an individual is guided. The athlete whose primary motivation is to gain an unfair advantage, or to prevent his or her opponent from gaining an unfair advantage, may be guided by his or her own moral principles and use performance-enhancing substances and thus violate the ethics underlying the Olympic ideal (Williams 1994).

Although no longer in effect, a previous section of the IOC doping rule read, in part, as follows: "Doping is the administration of or the use by a competing athlete of any ... physiological substance taken in abnormal quantity ... into the body, with the intention of increasing in an artificial and unfair manner his performance in competition" (Clark 1972). According to this stipulation, creatine supplementation could be regarded as doping. The doses that have been studied and that have been found to enhance performance approximate 20-30 g of creatine per day for 5 to 6 days. The best dietary sources of creatine are meat and fish, and in order to obtain 20-30 g from dietary sources, an athlete would need to consume about 7 kg of meat or fish. Although creatine is not foreign to the body and may be a normal constituent of the diet, an intake of 30 g would appear to contravene this aspect of the doping rule because the amount consumed may be abnormal in comparison to normal dietary intakes and may be taken with the primary intent of enhancing performance.

Contrasting viewpoints exist relative to the ethics of creatine supplementation. On the one hand, Greenhaff (1997a, 1997b) suggested that creatine could be viewed as an essential constituent of a "normal" diet and that creatine supplementation might augment muscle creatine stores in individuals low in endogenous creatine. Greenhaff also noted that creatine ingestion will increase muscle stores of this compound to no greater than their natural limit; therefore, ingestion could be considered to be no more malicious than the ingestion of large quantities of refined carbohydrate or glucose polymers, and it is difficult to see, given this, how creatine could become a banned substance. These viewpoints are supported by others, including Eric Hultman, the renowned Swedish physiologist, and Arne Ljungqvist, Chairman of the International Amateur Athletic Federation Medical Commission. Hultman indicates that creatine supplementation is no different than carbohydrate loading, hoping it can be a good alternative to drugs, while Ljungqvist compared supplementation with creatine to taking vitamin pills instead of vitamins in food (Associated Press 1993).

On the other hand, Maughan (1995) raises the ethical question whether the use of creatine should be disallowed on the grounds of its ergogenic effect, as is the case with other normal dietary components such as caffeine. The IOC permits athletes to consume small amounts of the stimulant caffeine because caffeine is a natural ingredient in several beverages and food products. However, large amounts of caffeine are prohibited, possibly because caffeine supplementation is regarded to be a very effective sport ergogenic. Nevertheless, even small amounts of caffeine permitted by the IOC may be powerful ergogenics (Graham and Spriet 1996; Spriet 1995). Maughan (1995) contends that there seems to be no logic to the argument for accepting the use of creatine in any dose while the amount of caffeine that may be used is restricted.

Contrasting viewpoints exist regarding the ethics of creatine supplementation. Some suggest that creatine could be viewed as an essential constituent of a "normal" diet, and that creatine supplementation might augment muscle creatine stores in individuals low in endogenous creatine. Others raise the ethical question whether the use of creatine should be disallowed on the grounds of its ergogenic effect, as is the case with other normal dietary components such as caffeine, a naturally occurring food drug.

Relative to the use of creatine supplementation as an ergogenic aid, both of the viewpoints described are logical. However, as creatine supplementation is not specifically prohibited by the IOC or other athletic governing organizations, its use by athletes should assumed to be ethical. In a sense, creatine supplementation is little different from other ergogenic techniques used by athletes, such as technological improvements in equipment to increase efficiency, psychological strategies to enhance mental strength, living in high-altitude houses to increase oxygen consumption, or even use of other nutrition-related supplements, such as alkaline or phosphate salts, that may be ergogenic.

As with any dietary supplement, whether marketed for health benefits or as a sport ergogenic, health professionals always express concern in relation to associated adverse health effects. Thus, because the long-term health effects of creatine supplementation are not completely understood at present, some contend that it may be unethical to recommend creatine supplementation to athletes or other physically active individuals.

Currently, under provisions of the DSHEA, the burden of proof of safety lies with the Food and Drug Administration, not the product manufacturer. Fortunately, when used as directed, the vast majority of dietary supplements are generally regarded as safe, and available research suggests that creatine is in this category. Epidemiological as well as experimental data do not indicate adverse health effects of short-term, 1-week loading protocols or of maintenance protocols for several months. However, there are very limited data regarding prolonged creatine supplementation, particularly with large dosages. Along these lines, athletes often believe that if one is good, then 10 is better, and may violate recommended protocols in attempts to increase the competitive edge.

Some researchers contend that it may be unethical to recommend creatine supplementation to athletes or other physically active individuals because the long-term health effects of creatine supplementation are not completely understood at present.

Based on the current ruling that creatine supplementation is legal, and on our current understanding regarding the health effects of creatine supplementation, the following recommendations would appear to be ethical. These recommendations are in accord with those for other dietary supplements, or even over-the-counter drugs.

- Individuals contemplating creatine supplementation should do so after being told of potential benefits and risks so that they may make an informed decision.
- Adolescent athletes involved in serious training should consider creatine supplementation only with approval and/or supervision of parents, trainers, coaches, and/or appropriate health professionals.
- Individuals should not exceed recommended doses. Research suggests that a creatine-loading protocol, approximately 20-30 g/day for 5 to 7 days, will maximize body stores of creatine.
- Maximal muscle creatine levels may be maintained with significantly lower daily doses of 2-5 g. There is no need to consume larger doses; larger amounts are not only more costly, but also ineffective.
- Athletic administrators in organized sports who wish to establish policies on creatine supplementation for teams should base such policies on the scientific literature. Any formal administration policy should be supervised by a qualified health professional.

Chapter Summary

Creatine, a natural dietary ingredient, has been classified as a food by the International Olympic Committee, and is legal for use by athletes. However, some contend that creatine supplementation falls in the gray zone between doping and substances allowed to enhance performance, linking its use to that of caffeine, a dietary ingredient and effective ergogenic aid whose use is banned when consumed in substantial amounts. Some also contend that it may be unethical to recommend creatine supplementation because the long-term health effects are not completely understood at present. However, current scientific data do not suggest that creatine supplementation, taken in recommended doses, poses any significant health risks. Nevertheless, individuals contemplating creatine supplementation should be aware of the possible risks, not exceed recommended dosages, and be under the guidance of trained health professionals where appropriate.

Bibliography

Aaserud, R., Gramvik, P., Olsen, S.R., and Jensen, J. 1998. Creatine supplementation delays onset of fatigue during repeated bouts of sprint running. *Scandinavian Journal of Medicine and Science in Sports* 8:247-251.

Almada, A., Kreider, R., Ferreira, M., Wilson, M., Grindstaff, P., Plisk, S., Reinhardy, J., and Cantler, E. 1997. Effects of calcium β-HMB supplementation with or without creatine during training on strength & sprint capacity. *FASEB Journal* 11: A374. (abstract).

Almada, A., Kreider, R., Weiss, L., Fry, A., Wood, L., Bullen, D., Miyaji, M., Grindstaff, P., Ramsey, L., and Li, Y. 1995. Effects of ingesting a supplement containing creatine monohydrate for 28 days on isokinetic performance. *Medicine and Science in Sports and Exercise* 27: S146. (abstract).

Almada, A., Mitchell, T., and Earnest, C. 1996. Impact of chronic creatine supplementation on serum enzyme concentrations. *FASEB Journal* 10: A791. (abstract).

Andrews, R., Greenhaff, P., Curtis, S., Perry, A., and Cowley, A.J. 1998. The effect of dietary creatine supplementation on skeletal muscle metabolism in congestive heart failure. *European Heart Journal* 19: 617-622.

Arias-Mendosa, F., Konchanin, L.M., Grover, W.D., Salganicoff, L., Selak, M.A., and Brown, T.R. 1998. Possible creatine synthesis deficit studied by in vivo magnetic resonance spectroscopy. *Medicine and Science in Sports and Exercise* 30: S234. (abstract).

Armour, S. 1998. Creatine: No scare just yet. *USA Today,* 24 April: Money, 1B.

Associated Press. 1993. Creatine naturally boosts performance. 9 May.

Associated Press. 1997a. Muscle building supplement to be investigated in wrestlers' deaths. 19 December.

Associated Press. 1997b. Wrestlers' deaths investigated. 11 December.

Associated Press. 1998a. FDA rejects creatine role in deaths. 30 April.

Associated Press. 1998b. McGwire riled by muscle drug story. 28 August.

Associated Press. 1998c. Soccer coach dismisses doping claim. 28 September.

Associated Press. 1998d. Wrestlers' deaths investigated. 14 January.

Associated Press. 1998e. New survey finds: Creatine use is high among athletes at all levels. 6 August.

Balsom, P.D., Ekblom, B., Söderlund, K., Sjödin, B., and Hultman, E. 1993a. Creatine supplementation and dynamic high-intensity intermittent exercise. *Scandinavian Journal of Medicine and Science in Sports* 3: 143-149.

Balsom, P.D., Harridge, S.D.R., Söderlund, K., Sjödin, B., and Ekblom, B. 1993b. Creatine supplementation per se does not enhance endurance exercise performance. *Acta Physiologica Scandinavica* 149: 521-523.

Balsom, P., Söderlund, K., and Ekblom, B. 1994. Creatine in humans with special reference to creatine supplementation. *Sports Medicine* 18: 268-280.

Balsom, P., Söderlund, K., Sjödin, B., and Ekblom, B. 1995. Skeletal muscle metabolism during short duration high-intensity exercise: Influence of creatine supplementation. *Acta Physiologica Scandinavica* 154: 303-310.

Bangsbo, J. 1994. Energy demands in competitive soccer. *Journal of Sports Science* 12: S5-S12.

Bangsbo, J., Gollnick, P.D., Graham, T.E., Juel, C., Kiens, B., Mizuno, M., and Saltin, B. 1990. Anaerobic energy production and O_2 deficit-debt relationship during exhaustive exercise in humans. *Journal of Physiology* 422: 539-559.

Barnett, C., Hinds, M., and Jenkins, D.G. 1996. Effects of oral creatine supplementation on multiple sprint cycle performance. *Australian Journal of Science and Medicine in Sports* 28: 35-39.

Becque, M.D., Lochmann, J.D., and Melrose, D. 1997. Effect of creatine supplementation during strength training on 1-RM and body composition. *Medicine and Science in Sports and Exercise* 29: S146. (abstract).

Bermon, S., Venembre, P., Sachet, C., Valour, S. and Dolisi, C. 1998. Effects of creatine monohydrate ingestion in sedentary and weight-trained older adults. *Acta Physiologica Scandinavica 164:* 146-155.

Bessman, S.P., and Mohan, C. 1992. Phosphocreatine, exercise, protein synthesis, and insulin. In *Guanidino compounds in biology and medicine,* ed. P.P. De Deyn, B. Maresceau, V. Statin, and I.A. Qureshi, pp. 181-186. London: John Libbey.

Bessman, S., and Savabi, F. 1988. The role of phosphocreatine energy shuttle in exercise and muscle hypertrophy. In *Creatine and creatine phosphate: Scientific and clinical perspectives,* ed. M.A. Conway and J.F. Clark, pp. 185-198. San Diego: Academic Press.

Birch, R., Nobel, D., and Greenhaff, P. 1994. The influence of dietary creatine supplementation on performance during repeated bouts of maximal isokinetic cycling in man. *European Journal of Applied Physiology* 69: 268-270.

Blei, M.L., Conley, K.E., and Kushmerick, M.J. 1993. Separate measures of ATP utilization and recovery in human skeletal muscle. *Journal of Physiology* 465: 203-222.

Bogdanis, G.C., Nevill, M.E., Boobis, L.H., Lakomy, H.K., and Nevill, A.M. 1995. Recovery of power output and muscle metabolites following 30 s of maximal sprint cycling in man. *Journal of Physiology* 482: 467-480.

Boicelli, C.A., Baldassarri, A.M., Borsetto, C., and Conconi, F. 1989. An approach to noninvasive fiber type determination by NMR. *International Journal of Sports Medicine* 10: 53-54.

Bolotte, C.P. 1998. Creatine supplementation in athletes: Benefits and potential risks. *Journal of the Louisiana State Medical Society*, 150: 325-327.

Bosco, C., Tihanyi, J., Pucspk, J., Kovacs, I., Gabossy, A., Colli, R., Puivirenti, G., Tranquilli, C., Foti, C., Viru, M., and Viru, A. 1997. Effect of oral creatine supplementation on jumping and running performance. *International Journal of Sports Medicine* 18: 369-372.

Bosco, C., Tranquilli, C., Tihanyi, J., Colli, R., D'Ottavio, S., and Viru, A. 1995. Influence of oral supplementation with creatine monohydrate on physical capacity evaluated in laboratory and field tests. *Medinca dello Sport* 48: 391-397.

Brannon, T.A., Adams, G.R., Conniff, C.L., and Baldwin, K.M. 1997. Effects of creatine loading and training on running performance and biochemical properties of rat skeletal muscle. *Medicine and Science in Sports and Exercise* 29: 489-495.

Brees, A.J., Cordain, L., Harris, M., Smith, M.J., Fahrney, D., Gotshall, R., and Devoe, D. 1994. Creatine ingestion does not influence leg extension power in meat eating and vegetarian females. *FASEB Journal* 8:A308 (abstract).

Burke, L.M., Pyne, D.B., and Telford, R.D. 1996. Effect of oral creatine supplementation on single-effort sprint performance in elite swimmers. *International Journal of Sport Nutrition* 6: 222-233.

Casey, A., Constantin-Teodosiu, D., Howell, S., Hultman, E., and Greenhaff, P.L. 1996. Creatine ingestion favorably affects performance and muscle metabolism during maximal exercise in humans. *American Journal of Physiology* 271: E31-E37.

Cerretelli, P., and diPrampero, P.E. 1987. Gas exchange in exercise. In *Handbook of physiology, Section 3: The respiratory system, Vol. IV: Gas exchange,* ed. A.P. Fishman, L.E. Farhi, S.M. Tenney and S.R. Geiger, pp. 297-339. Bethesda, MD: American Physiological Society.

Chanutin, A. 1926. The fate of creatine when administered to man. *Journal of Biological Chemistry* 67: 29-41.

Chetlin, R., Schoenleber, J., Bryner, R., Gordon, P., Ullrich, I., and Yeater, R. 1998. The effects of two forms of oral creatine supplementation on anaerobic performance during the Wingate test. *Journal of Strength and Conditioning Research* 12: 273. (abstract).

Clark, J.F. 1996. *Uses of creatine phosphate and creatine supplementation for the athlete.* In creatine and creatine phosphate: scientific and clinical perspectives, ed. M.A. Conway and J.F. Clark, pp. 217-226. San Diego: Academic Press.

Clark, J.F. 1997. Creatine and phosphocreatine: A review of their use in exercise and sport. *Journal of Athletic Training* 32: 45-50.

Clark, J.F. 1998. Creatine: A review of its nutritional applications in sport. *Nutrition* 14: 322-324.

Clark, J.F., Field, M.L., and Ventura-Clapier, R. 1996a. An introduction to the cellular creatine kinase system in contractile tissue. In *Creatine and creatine phosphate: Scientific and clinical perspectives,* ed. M.A. Conway and J.F. Clark, pp. 51-64. San Diego: Academic Press.

Clark, J.F., Odoom, J., Tracey, I., Dunn, J., Boehm, E.A., Paternostro, G., and Radda, G.K. 1996b. Experimental observations of creatine and creatine phosphate metabolism. In *Creatine and creatine phosphate: Scientific and clinical perspectives,* ed. M.A. Conway and J.F. Clark, pp. 33-50. San Diego: Academic Press.

Clark, K. 1972. *Drugs and the coach,* p. 28. Washington, DC: American Alliance for Health, Physical Education, and Recreation.

Constantin-Teodosiu, D., Greenhaff, P.L., Gardiner, S.M., Randall, M.D., March, J.E., and Bennett, T. 1995. Attenuation by creatine of myocardial metabolic stress in Brattleboro rats caused by chronic inhibition of nitric oxide synthase. *British Journal of Pharmacology* 116: 3288-3292.

Conway, M.A., and Clark, J.F., eds. 1996a. *Creatine and creatine phosphate: Scientific and clinical perspectives.* San Diego: Academic Press.

Conway, M.A., and Clark, J.F. 1996b. Creatine and creatine phosphate: Future perspectives. In *Creatine and creatine phosphate: Scientific and clinical perspectives,* ed. M.A. Conway and J.F. Clark, pp. 227-229. San Diego: Academic Press.

Conway, M.A., Ouwerkerk, R., Rajagopalan, B., and Radda, G.K. 1996a. Creatine phosphate: In vivo human cardiac metabolism studied by magnetic resonance spectroscopy. In *Creatine and creatine phosphate: Scientific and clinical perspectives,* ed. M.A. Conway and J.F. Clark, pp. 127-159. San Diego: Academic Press.

Conway, M.A., Rajagopalan, B., and Radda, G.K. 1996b. Skeletal muscle metabolism in heart failure. In *Creatine and creatine phosphate: Scientific and clinical perspectives,* ed. M.A. Conway and J.F. Clark, pp. 162-182. San Diego: Academic Press.

Cooke, W.H., and Barnes, W.S. 1997. The influence of recovery duration on high-intensity exercise performance after oral creatine supplementation. *Canadian Journal of Applied Physiology* 22: 454-467.

Cooke, W.H., Grandjean, P.W., and Barnes, W.S. 1995. Effect of oral creatine supplementation on power output and fatigue during bicycle ergometry. *Journal of Applied Physiology* 78: 670-673.

Costley, C.D., Mandel, C.H., and Schwenck, T.L. 1998. Nutritional supplement use in collegiate athletes. *Medicine and Science in Sports and Exercise* 30: S40. (abstract).

Cowan, D.A. 1997. Testing for drug abuse. In *The clinical pharmacology of sport and exercise,* ed. T. Reilly and M. Orme, pp. 13-23. Amsterdam: Elsevier Science.

Crim, M.C., Calloway, D.H., and Margen, S. 1975. Creatine metabolism in men: Urinary creatine and creatinine excretions with creatine feedings. *Journal of Nutrition* 105: 428-438.

Crim, M.C., Calloway, D.H., and Margen, S. 1976. Creatine metabolism in men: Creatine pool size and turnover in relation to creatine intake. *Journal of Nutrition* 106: 371-381.

Crowder, T., Jensen, N., Richmond, S., Voigts, J., Sweeney, B., McIntyre, G., and Thompson, B. 1998. Influence of creatine type and diet on strength and body composition of collegiate lightweight football players. *Medicine and Science in Sports and Exercise* 30: S264. (abstract).

Dawson, B., Cutler, M., Moody, A., Lawrence, S., Goodman, C., and Randall, N. 1995. Effects of oral creatine loading on single and repeated maximal short sprints. *Australian Journal of Science and Medicine in Sports* 27: 56-61.

Delanghe, J., De Slypere, J.P., De Buyzere, M., Robbrecht, J., Wieme, R., and Vermeulen, A. 1989. Normal reference values for creatine, creatinine, and carnitine are lower in vegetarians. *Clinical Chemistry* 35: 1802-1803.

Dixon, O. 1998. CWS coaches say creatine a factor. *USA Today,* 29 May: Sports, C3.

Duarte, J. 1998. For athletes, potion has powerful lure. *Houston Chronicle,* 13 March, 1A, 14A.

Earnest, C.P., Almada, A.L., and Mitchell, T.L. 1996a. High-performance capillary electrophoresis-pure creatine monohydrate reduced blood lipids in men and women. *Clinical Science* 91: 113-118.

Earnest, C.P., Almada, A.L., and Mitchell, T.L. 1996b. Influence of chronic creatine supplementation on hepatorenal function. *FASEB Journal* 10: A790. (abstract).

Earnest, C.P., Snell, P.G., Rodriguez, R., Almada, A.L., and Mitchell, T.L. 1995. The effect of creatine monohydrate ingestion on anaerobic power indices, muscular strength and body composition. *Acta Physiologica Scandinavica* 153: 207-209.

Earnest, C.P., Almada, A.L., and Mitchell, T.L. 1997. Effects of creatine monohydrate ingestion on intermediate duration anaerobic treadmill running to exhaustion. *Journal of Strength and Conditioning Research* 11: 234-238.

Earnest, C.P., Beckham, S., and Whyte, B.O. 1998. Effect of acute creatine ingestion on anaerobic performance. *Medicine and Science in Sports and Exercise* 30: S141. (abstract).

Ekblom, B. 1996. Effects of creatine supplementation on performance. *American Journal of Sports Medicine* 24: S38-S39.

Engelhardt, M., Neumann, G., Berbalk, A., and Reuter, I. 1998. Creatine supplementation in endurance sports. *Medicine and Science in Sports and Exercise* 30: 1123-1129.

Ensign, W.Y., Jacobs, I., Prusaczyk, W.K., Goforth, H.W., Law, P.G., and Schneider, K.E. 1998. Effects of creatine supplementation on short-term anaerobic exercise performance of U.S. Navy Seals. *Medicine and Science in Sports and Exercise* 30: S265. (abstract).

Ferraro, S., Codella, C., Palumbo, F., Desiderio, A., Trimigliozzi, P., Maddalena, G., and Chiariello, M. (1996). Hemodynamic effects of creatine phosphate in patients with congestive heart failure: A double-blind comparison trial versus placebo. *Clinical Cardiology*, 19:699-703.

Febbraio, M.A., Flanagan, T.R., Snow, R.J., Zhao, S., and Carey, M.F. 1995. Effect of creatine supplementation on intramuscular TCr, metabolism and performance during intermittent, supramaximal exercise in humans. *Acta Physiologica Scandinavica* 155: 387-395.

Fogelholm, M., and Saris, W.H.M. 1998. Making weight for sports participation. In *Oxford textbook of sports medicine,* ed. M. Harries, C. Williams, W.D. Stanish, and L.J. Micheli, pp. 113-126. Oxford: Oxford University Press.

Francaux, M., and Poortmans, J.R. 1999. Effects of training and creatine supplement on muscle strength and body mass. *European Journal of Applied Physiology*: In press.

Gilliam, J.D., Hohzom, C., and Martin, A.D. 1998. Effect of oral creatine supplementation on isokinetic force production. *Medicine and Science in Sports and Exercise* 30: S140. (abstract).

Godly, A., and Yates, J.W. 1997. Effects of creatine supplementation on endurance cycling combined with short, high-intensity bouts. *Medicine and Science in Sports and Exercise* 29: S251. (abstract).

Gola, H. 1998. Thousands turn to creatine to bulk up bodies. *Knight-Ridder Newspaper,* 22 April.

Goldberg, P.G., and Bechtel, P.J. 1997. Effects of low dose creatine supplementation on strength, speed and power events by male athletes. *Medicine and Science in Sports and Exercise* 29: S251. (abstract).

Gonzalez de Suso, J.M., Moreno, A., Francaux, M., Alonso, J., Porta, J., Font, J., Arus, C., and Prat, J.A. 1995. [31] P-MRS detects an increase in muscle phosphocreatine content after oral creatine supplementation in trained subjects. *Third IOC World Congress on Sports Sciences Congress Proceedings,* p. 347. Atlanta: Xerox Docutech 135 Network Publishers. (abstract).

Gonzalez de Suso, J.M., and Prat, J.A. 1994. Dietary supplementation using orally-taken creatine monohydrate in humans. *CAR News* 6: 4-9.

Gordon, A., Hultman, E., Kaijser, L., Kristjansson, S., Rolf, C.J., Nyquist, O., and Sylven, C. 1995. Creatine supplementation in chronic heart failure increases skeletal muscle creatine phosphate and muscle performance. *Cardiovascular Research* 30: 413-438.

Graham, T., and Spriet, L. 1996. Caffeine and exercise performance. *Sports Science Exchange* 9(1): 1-5.

Green, A.L., Greenhaff, P.L., MacDonald, I.A., Bell, D., Holliman, D., and Stroud, M.A. 1993. The influence of oral creatine supplementation on metabolism during sub-maximal incremental treadmill exercises. *Proceedings of the Nutrition Society*, 53:84A. (abstract).

Green, A.L., Hultman, E., MacDonald, I.A., Sewell, D.A., and Greenhaff, P.L. 1996a. Carbohydrate feeding augments skeletal muscle creatine accumulation during creatine supplementation in humans. *American Journal of Physiology* 271: E821-E826.

Green, A.L., Simpson, E.J., Littlewood, J.J., MacDonald, I.A., and Greenhaff, P.L. 1996b. Carbohydrate ingestion augments creatine retention during creatine feeding in humans. *Acta Physiologica Scandinavica* 158: 195-202.

Greenhaff, P.L. 1995. Creatine and its application as an ergogenic aid. *International Journal of Sport Nutrition* 5: S100-S110.

Greenhaff, P.L. 1998. Renal dysfunction accompanying oral creatine supplements. *Lancet* 352: 233-234.

Greenhaff, P.L. 1996. Creatine supplementation: Recent developments. *British Journal of Sports Medicine* 30: 276-277.

Greenhaff, P.L. 1997a. Creatine supplementation and implications for exercise performance and guidelines for creatine supplementation. In *Advances in training and nutrition for endurance sports,* ed. A. Jeukendrup, M. Brouns, and F. Brouns. Maastricht: Novartis Nutrition Research Unit. January 30: 8-11.

Greenhaff, P.L. 1997b. The nutritional biochemistry of creatine. *Journal of Nutritional Biochemistry* 11: 610-618.

Greenhaff, P.L., Bodin, K., Harris, R.C., Hultman, E., Jones, D.A., McIntyre, D.B., Söderlund, K., and Turner, D.L. 1993a. The influence of oral creatine supplementation on muscle phosphocreatine resynthesis following intense contraction in man. *Journal of Physiology* 467: 75P. (abstract).

Greenhaff, P.L., Bodin, K., Söderlund, K., and Hultman, E. 1994a. Effect of oral creatine supplementation on skeletal muscle phosphocreatine resynthesis. *American Journal of Physiology* 266: E725-E730. (abstract).

Greenhaff, P.L., Casey, A., and Green, A. 1996. Creatine supplementation revisited: An update. *Insider* 4(3): 1-2.

Greenhaff, P.L., Casey, A., Short, A.H., Harris, R., Söderlund, K., and Hultman, E. 1993b. Influence of oral creatine supplementation of [sic] muscle torque during repeated bouts of maximal voluntary exercise in man. *Clinical Science* 84: 565-571.

Greenhaff, P.L., Constantin-Teodosiu, D., Casey, A., and Hultman, E. 1994b. The effect of oral creatine supplementation on skeletal muscle ATP degradation during repeated bouts of maximal voluntary exercise in man. *Journal of Physiology* 476: 84P. (abstract).

Greenhaff, P.L., Nevill, M.E., Söderlund, K., Boobis, L., Williams, C., and Hultman, E. 1992. Energy metabolism in single muscle fibres during maximal sprint exercise in man. *Journal of Physiology* 446: 528P. (abstract).

Grindstaff, P., Kreider, R., Weiss, L., Fry, A., Wood, L., Bullen, D., Miyaji, M., Ramsey, L., Li, Y., and Almada, A. 1995. Effects of ingesting a supplement containing creatine monohydrate for 7 days on isokinetic performance. *Medicine and Science in Sports and Exercise* 27: S146. (abstract).

Grindstaff, P.D., Kreider, R., Bishop, R., Wilson, M., Wood, L., Alexander, C., and Almada, A. 1997. Effects of creatine supplementation on repetitive sprint performance and body composition in competitive swimmers. *International Journal of Sport Nutrition* 7: 330-346.

Grunewald, K., and Bailey, R. 1993. Commercially marketed supplements for bodybuilding athletes. *Sports Medicine* 15: 90-103.

Guerrero-Ontiveros, M.L., and Wallimann, T. 1998. Creatine supplementation in health and disease. Effects of chronic creatine ingestion in vivo: Down-regulation of the expression of creatine transporter isoforms in skeletal muscle. *Molecular and Cellular Biochemistry* 184: 427-437.

Hamilton-Ward, K., Meyers, M.C., Skelly, W.A., Marley, R.J., and Saunders, J. 1997. Effect of creatine supplementation on upper extremity anaerobic response in females. *Medicine and Science in Sports and Exercise* 29: S146. (abstract).

Harris, R.C., Söderlund, K., and Hultman, E. 1992. Elevation of creatine in resting and exercised muscle of normal subjects by creatine supplementation. *Clinical Science* 83: 367-374.

Haughland, R.B., and Chang, D.T. 1975. Insulin effects on creatine transport in skeletal muscle. *Proceedings of the Society of Experimental Biology and Medicine* 148: 1-4.

Häussinger, D., Roth, E., Lang, F., and Gerok, W. 1993. Cellular hydration state: An important determinant of protein catabolism in health and disease. *Lancet* 341: 1330-1332.

Hawley, J.A., Schabort, E.B., Noakes, T.D., and Dennis, J.C. 1997. Carbohydrate loading and exercise performance. *Sports Medicine* 24: 73-81.

Hellmich, N. 1998a. No link found to creatine in 3 student deaths. *USA Today,* 30 April, D1.

Hellmich, N. 1998b. Safety still a creatine issue. *USA Today,* 4 June, C3.

Hirvonen, J., Rehunen, S., Rusko, H., and Harkonen, M. 1987. Breakdown of high-energy phosphate compounds and lactate accumulation during short supramaximal exercise. *European Journal of Applied Physiology* 56: 253-259.

Hoberman, H.D., Sims, E.A., and Peters, J.H. 1948. Creatine and creatinine metabolism in the normal male adult studied with the aid of isotopic nitrogen. *Journal of Biological Chemistry* 172: 45-51.

Hochachka, P.W. 1994. *Muscles as molecular and metabolic machines.* Boca Raton, FL: CRC Press.

Horn, M., Frantz, S., Remkes, H., Laser, A., Urban, B., Mettenleiter, A., Schnackerz, K., and Neubauer, S. 1998. Effects of chronic dietary creatine feeding on cardiac energy metabolism and on creatine content in heart, skeletal muscle, brain, liver and kidney. *Journal of Molecular and Cellular Cardiology* 30: 277-284.

Hultman, E., and Greenhaff, P.L. 1991. Skeletal muscle energy metabolism and fatigue during intense exercise in man. *Science Progress* 75(298, Part 3-4): 361-370.

Hultman, E., Greenhaff, P.L., Rem, J.M., and Söderlund, K. 1991. Energy metabolism and fatigue during intense muscle contraction. *Biochemical Society Transactions* 19: 347-353.

Hultman, E., and Sahlin, K. 1980. Acid-base balance during exercise. *Exercise and Sports Science Reviews* 8: 41-128.

Hultman, E., Söderland, K., Timmons, J.A., Cederblad, G., and Greenhaff, P.L. 1996. Muscle creatine loading in men. *Journal of Applied Physiology* 81: 232-237.

Hunt, J., Kreider, R., Melton, C., Ransom, J., Rasmussen, C., Stroud, T., Cantler, E., and Milnor, P. 1999. Creatine does not increase incidence of cramping or injury during pre-season college football training II. *Medicine and Science in Sports and Exercise* 31(5): in press.

Hunter, A. 1928. *Monographs on biochemistry: Creatine and creatinine.* London: Longmans, Green.

Ingwall, J.S. 1976. Creatine and the control of muscle-specific protein synthesis in cardiac and skeletal muscle. *Circulation Research* 38: I-115-I-123.

Ingwall, J.S., Morales, M.F., and Stockdale, F.E. 1972. Creatine and the control of myosin synthesis in differentiating skeletal muscle. *Proceedings of the National Academy of Sciences* 69: 2250-2253.

Ingwall, J.S., Weiner, C.D., Morales, M.F., Davis, E., and Stockdale, F.E. 1974. Specificity of creatine in the control of muscle protein synthesis. *Journal of Cellular Biology* 63: 145-151.

Irving, R.A., Noakes, T.D., Burger, S.C., Myburgh, K.H., Querido, D., and van Zyl-Smit, R. 1990. Plasma volume and renal function during and after ultramarathon running. *Medicine and Science in Sports and Exercise* 22: 581-587.

Irving, R.A., Noakes, T.D., Irving, G.A., and van Zyl-Smit, R. 1986. The immediate and delayed effects of marathon running on renal function. *Journal of Urology* 136: 1176-1180.

Jacobs, I., Bleue, S., and Goodman, J. 1997. Creatine ingestion increases anaerobic capacity and maximal accumulated oxygen deficit. *Canadian Journal of Applied Physiology* 22: 231-243.

Janssen, G.M., Degenaar, C.P., Menheere, P.P., Habets, H.M., and Geurten, P. 1989. Plasma urea, creatinine, uric acid, albumin, and total protein concentrations before and after 15-, 25- and 42-km contests. *International Journal of Sports Medicine* 10: S132-S138.

Javierre, C., Lizarraga, M.A., Ventura, J.L., Garrido, E., and Segura, R. 1997. Creatine supplementation does not improve physical performance in a 150 m race. *Revista Espanola de Fisiologia* 53: 343-348.

Johnson, K.D., Smodic, B., and Hill, R. 1997. The effects of creatine monohydrate supplementation on muscular power and work. *Medicine and Science in Sports and Exercise* 29: S251. (abstract).

Johnson, R. 1998. Demographics of creatine monohydrate users. Memorandum to Brett Hall, *Experimental and Applied Sciences*, 30 July.

Jones, A.M., Atter, T., and George, K.P. 1998. Oral creatine supplementation improves multiple sprint performance in elite ice-hockey players. *Medicine and Science in Sports and Exercise* 30: S140. (abstract).

Juhn, M.S., and Tarnopolsky, M. 1998a. Oral creatine supplementation and athletic performance: A critical review. *Clinical Journal of Sport Medicine*. 8: 286-297.

Juhn, M.S., and Tarnopolsky, M. 1998b. Potential side effects of oral creatine supplementation: A critical review. *Clinical Journal of Sport Medicine*. 8: 298-304.

Kamber, M., Koster, M., Kreis, R., Walker, G., Boesch, C., and Hoppebee, H. 1999. Creatine Supplementation. Part I. Performance, clinical chemistry and muscle volume. *Medicine and Science in Sports and Exercise.* In Press.

Kargotich, S., Goodman, C., Keast, D., Fry, R.W., Garcia-Webb, P., Crawford, P.M., and Morton, A.R. 1997. Influence of exercise-induced plasma volume changes on the interpretation of biochemical data following high-intensity exercise. *Clinical Journal of Sports Medicine* 7: 185-191.

Katz, A., Sahlin, K., and Henriksson, J. 1986. Muscle ATP turnover rate during isometric contraction in humans. *Journal of Applied Physiology* 60: 1839-1842.

Kelly, V.G., and Jenkins, D.G. 1998. Effect of oral creatine supplementation on near-maximal strength and repeated sets of high-intensity bench press exercise. *Journal of Strength and Conditioning Research* 12: 109-115.

Kent-Braun, J.A., Sharma, K.R., Miller, R.G., and Weiner, M.W. 1994. Post-exercise phosphocreatine resynthesis is slowed in multiple sclerosis. *Muscle and Nerve* 17: 835-841.

Khanna, N.K., and Madan, B.R. 1978. Studies on the anti-inflammatory activity of creatine. *Archives Internationales de Pharmacodynamie* 231: 340-350.

Kirksey, K.B., Warren, B.J., Stone, M.H., Stone, M.R., and Johnson, R.L. 1997. The effects of six weeks of creatine monohydrate supplementation in male and female track athletes. *Medicine and Science in Sports and Exercise* 29: S145. (abstract).

Knehans, A., Bemben, M., Bemben, D., and Loftiss, D. 1998. Creatine supplementation affects body composition and neuromuscular performance in football athletes. *FASEB Journal* 12: A863. (abstract).

Kraemer, W.J., and Volek, J.S. 1998. Creatine supplementation: Current comment from the American College of Sports Medicine. Indianapolis: American College of Sports Medicine.

Kreider, R., Ferreira, M., Wilson, M., and Almada, A. 1997a. Effects of creatine supplementation with and without glucose on body composition in trained and untrained men and women. *Journal of Strength and Conditioning Research* 11: 283. (abstract).

Kreider, R., Ferreira, M., Wilson, M., and Almada, A. 1998a. Effects of creatine supplementation with and without glucose on repetitive sprint performance in trained and untrained men and women. *International Journal of Sport Nutrition* 8: 204-205. (abstract).

Kreider, R., Ferreira, M., Wilson, M., Grindstaff, P., Plisk, S., Reinhardy, J., Cantler, E., and Almada, A. 1997b. Effects of ingesting a supplement designed to enhance creatine uptake on body composition during training. *Medicine and Science in Sports and Exercise* 29: S145. (abstract).

Kreider, R., Ferreira, M., Wilson, M., Grindstaff, P., Plisk, S., Reinhardy, J., Cantler, E., and Almada, A. 1998b. Effects of creatine supplementation on body composition, strength, and sprint performance. *Medicine and Science in Sports and Exercise* 30: 73-82.

Kreider, R., Grindstaff, P., Wood, L., Bullen, D., Klesges, R., Lotz, D., Davis, M., Cantler, E., and Almada, A. 1996a. Effects of ingesting a lean mass promoting supplement during resistance training on isokinetic performance. *Medicine and Science in Sports and Exercise* 28: S36. (abstract).

Kreider, R., Melton, C., Hunt, C., Rasmussen, C., Ransom, J., Stroud, T., Cantler, E., and Milnor, P. 1999a. Creatine does not increase incidence of cramping or injury during pre-season college football training I. *Medicine and Science in Sports and Exercise* 31(5): in press. (abstract).

Kreider, R., Ransom, J., Rasmussen, C., Hunt, C., Melton, C., Stroud, T., Cantler, E., and Milnor, P. 1999b. Creatine supplementation during pre-season football training does not affect markers of renal function. *FASEB Journal* 13: in press. (abstract).

Kreider, R., Rasmussen, C., Ransom, J., and Almada, A. 1998c. Effects of creatine supplementation during training on the incidence of muscle cramping, injuries and GI distress. *Journal of Strength and Conditioning Research* 12: 275. (abstract).

Kreider, R., Rasmussen, C., Ransom, J., Melton, C., Hunt, J., Almada, A.L., Tutko, R., and Milnor, P. 1999c. Relationship between creatine supplementation history and markers of clinical status in college football players. Southeast American College of Sports Medicine conference abstracts. 27: 30. (abstract).

Kreider, R., Wood, L., Bullen, D., Grindstaff, P., and Almada, A. 1995. Effects of ingesting a supplement containing creatine monohydrate on isokinetic performance. *Journal of Strength and Conditioning Research* 9: 282-283. (abstract).

Kreider, R.B. 1998a. Creatine supplementation: Analysis of ergogenic value, medical safety, and concerns. *Journal of Exercise Physiology*$_{online}$ 1: 7-18. **http://www.css.edu/users/ tboone2/asep/jan3.htm.**

Kreider, R.B. 1998b. Creatine, the next ergogenic supplement? In Sport Science Training and Technology, Internet Society for Sport Science. **http://www.sportsci.org/traintech/creatine/rbk.html.**

Kreider, R.B., Klesges, R., Harmon, K., Grindstaff, P., Ramsey, L., Bullen, D., Wood, L., Li, Y., and Almada, A. 1996b. Effects of ingesting supplements designed to promote lean tissue accretion on body composition during resistance training. *International Journal of Sport Nutrition* 6: 234-246.

Kreis, R., Koster, M., Kambler, M., Hoppeler, H., and Boesch, C. 1997. Peak assignment in localized 1h MR spectra of human muscle based on oral creatine supplementation. *Magnetic Resonance Medicine* 37: 159-163.

Kuehl, K., Goldberg, L., and Elliot, D. 1998. Renal insufficiency after creatine supplementation in a college football athlete. *Medicine and Science in Sports and Exercise* 30: S235. (abstract).

Kurosawa, Y., Iwane, H., Hamaoka, T., Shimomitsu, T., Katsumura, T., Sako, T., Kuwamori, M., and Kimura, N. 1997. Effects of oral creatine supplementation on high- and low-intensity grip exercise performance. *Medicine and Science in Sports and Exercise* 29: S251. (abstract).

Kurosawa, Y., Katsumura, T., Hamaoka, T., Kuwamori, M., Sako, T., Kimura, N., and Shimomitsu, T. 1998a. Effects of oral creatine supplementation on muscle oxidative capacity during dynamic grip exercise. *Medicine and Science in Sports and Exercise* 30: S141. (abstract).

Kurosawa, Y., Katsumura, T., Hamaoka, T., Sako, T., Iwane, H., Kuwamori, M., Kimura, N., and Shimomitsu, T. 1998b. Effects of oral creatine supplementation on localized muscle performance and muscle creatine phosphate concentration. *Japanese Journal of Physical Fitness and Sports Medicine* 47: 361-366.

Larson, D.E., Hunter, G.R., Trowbridge, C.A., Turk, J.C., Harbin, P.A., and Torman, S.L. 1998. Creatine supplementation and performance during off-season training in female soccer players. *Medicine and Science in Sports and Exercise* 30: S264. (abstract).

Lawson, E., Lemon, P., Volek, J., Stone, M., and Kreider, R. 1998. Creatine: Scientific information and practical guidelines. National Strength and Conditioning Association Pre-Conference Symposia, Nashville, TN, June 24.

Ledford, A., and Branch, J.D. 1999. Creatine supplementation does not increase peak power production and work capacity during repetitive Wingate testing in women. *Journal of Strength and Conditioning Research.* In press.

Leenders, N., Sherman, W.M., Lamb, D.R., and Nelson, T.E. 1999. Creatine supplementation and swimming performance. *International Journal of Sport Nutrition.* 9: In press.

Leenders, N., Lesniewski, L.A., Sherman, W.M., Sand, G., Sand, S., Mulroy, S., and Lamb, D.R. 1996. Dietary creatine supplementation and swimming performance. *Overtraining and Overreaching in Sports Conference Abstracts* 1: 80.

Lefavi, R.G., McMillan, J.L., Kahn, P.J., Crosby, J.F., Digioacchino, R.F., and Streater, J.A. 1998. Effects of creatine monohydrate on performance of collegiate baseball and basketball players. *Journal of Strength and Conditioning Research* 12: 275. (abstract).

Lemon, P., Boska, M., Bredle, D., Rogers, M., Ziegenfuss, T., and Newcomer, B. 1995. Effect of oral creatine supplementation on energetics during repeated maximal muscle contraction. *Medicine and Science in Sports and Exercise* 27: S204. (abstract).

Loike, J.D., Zalutsky, D.L., Kaback, E., Miranda, A.F., and Silverstein, S.C. 1988. Extracellular creatine regulates creatine transport in rat and human muscle cells. *Proceedings of the National Academy of Sciences* 85: 807-811.

Long, D., Blake, M., McNaughton, L., and Angle, B. 1990. Hematological and biochemical changes during a short triathlon competition in novice triathletes. *European Journal of Applied Physiology* 61: 93-99.

Ma, T.M., Friedman, D.L., and Roberts, R. 1996. Creatine phosphate shuttle pathway in tissues with dynamic energy demand. In *Creatine and creatine phosphate: Scientific and clinical perspectives,* ed. M.A. Conway and J.F. Clark, pp. 17-32. San Diego: Academic Press.

Maganaris, C.N., and Maughan, R.J. 1998. Creatine supplementation enhances maximum voluntary isometric force and endurance capacity in resistance trained men. *Acta Physiologica Scandinavica* 163: 279-287.

Mahler, M. 1980. Kinetics and control of oxygen consumption in skeletal muscle. In *Symposia of the Giovanni Lorenzini Foundation, Vol. 9: Exercise bioenergetics and gas exchange,* ed. P. Cerretelli and B.J. Whipp, pp. 53-66. Amsterdam: Elsevier/North-Holland Biomedical Press.

Matthews, R.T., Yang, L., Jenkins, B.G., Ferrante, R.J., Rosen, B.R., Kaddurah-Daouk, R., and Beal, M.F. 1998. Neuroprotective effects of creatine and cyclocreatine in animal models of Huntington's disease. *Journal of Neuroscience* 18: 156-163.

Maughan, R.J. 1995. Creatine supplementation and exercise performance. *International Journal of Sport Nutrition* 5: 94-101.

McCully, K.K., Vandenborne, K., DeMeirleir, K., Posner, J.D., and Leigh, J.S. 1992. Muscle metabolism in track athletes, using ^{31}P magnetic resonance spectroscopy. *Canadian Journal of Physiology and Pharmacology* 70: 1353-1359.

McNaughton, L.R., Dalton, B., and Tarr, J. 1998. The effects of creatine supplementation on high-intensity exercise performance in elite performers. *European Journal of Applied Physiology* 78: 236-240.

Melton, C., Kreider, R., Rasmussen, J., Ransom, J., Hunt, J., Stroud, E., Cantler, E., and Milnor, P. 1999. Effects of ingesting creatine containing supplements during training on blood lipid profiles. *FASEB Journal* 13: in press. (abstract).

Mihic, S., MacDonald, J.R., McKenzie, S., and Tarnopolsky, M.A. 1998. The effect of creatine supplementation on blood pressure, plasma creatine kinase, and body composition. *FASEB Journal* 12: A652. (abstract).

Mihoces, G. 1998. The theory behind the supplement's use. *USA Today,* 23 April: Money, 2B.

Miller, E.E., Evans, A.E., and Cohn, M. 1993. Inhibition of rate of tumor growth by creatine and cyclocreatine. *Proceedings of the National Academy of Sciences* 90: 3304-3308.

Miller, R.G., Boska, M.D., Moussavi, R.S., Carson, P.J., and Weiner, M.W. 1988. ^{31}P nuclear magnetic resonance studies of high energy phosphates and pH in human muscle fatigue. Comparison of aerobic and anaerobic exercise. *Journal of Clinical Investigation* 81: 1190-1196.

Miller, R.G., Giannini, D., Milner-Brown, H.S., Layzer, R.B., Koretsky, A.P., Hooper, D., and Weiner, M.W. 1987. Effects of fatiguing exercise on high-energy phosphates, force, and EMG: Evidence for three phases of recovery. *Muscle and Nerve* 10: 810-821.

Miszko, T.A., Baer, J.T., and Vanderbergh, P.M. 1998. The effect of creatine loading on body mass and vertical jump of female athletes. *Medicine and Science in Sports and Exercise* 30: S141. (abstract).

Mujika, I., Chatard, J.C., Lacoste, L., Barale, F., and Geyssant, A. 1996. Creatine supplementation does not improve sprint performance in competitive swimmers. *Medicine and Science in Sports and Exercise* 28: 1435-1441.

Mujika, I., and Padilla, S. 1997. Creatine supplementation as an ergogenic aid for sports performance in highly trained athletes: A critical review. *International Journal of Sports Medicine* 18: 491-496.

Myburgh, K.H., Bold, A., Bellinger, B., Wilson, G., and Noakes, T.D. 1996. Creatine supplementation and sprint training in cyclists: Metabolic and performance effects. *Medicine and Science in Sports and Exercise* 28: S81. (abstract).

Nelson, A., Day, R., Glickman-Weiss, E., Hegstad, M., and Sampson, B. 1997. Creatine supplementation raises anaerobic threshold. *FASEB Journal* 11: A589. (abstract).

Newsholme, E.A., and Beis, I. 1996. Old and new ideas on the roles of phosphagens and their kinases. In *Creatine and creatine phosphate: Scientific and clinical perspectives,* ed. M.A. Conway and J.F. Clark, pp. 3-15. San Diego: Academic Press.

Noonan, B., French, J., and Street, G. 1998a. Creatine supplementation and multiple skating task performance in Division I hockey players. *Medicine and Science in Sports and Exercise* 30: S310. (abstract).

Noonan, D., Berg, K., Latin, R.W., Wagner, J.C., and Reimers, K. 1998b. Effects of varying dosages of oral creatine relative to fat free body mass on strength and body composition. *Journal of Strength and Conditioning Research* 12: 104-108.

Odland, L.M., MacDougall, J.D., Tarnopolsky, M.A., Elorriaga, A., Borgmann, A., and Atkinson, S. 1997. Effect of oral creatine supplementation on muscle [PCr] and short-term maximum power output. *Medicine and Science in Sports and Exercise* 29: 216-219.

O'Donnell, J., and Mihoces, G. 1998. FDA warning out on sports supplement. *USA Today,* 23 April: News, 1A.

Ööpik, V., Pääsuke, M., Timpmann, S., Medijainen, L., Ereline, J., and Smirnova, T. 1998. Effect of creatine supplementation during rapid body mass reduction on metabolism and isokinetic muscle performance capacity. *European Journal of Applied Physiology* 78: 83-92.

Ööpik, V., Timpmann, S., and Medijainen, L. 1995. The role and application of dietary creatine supplementation in increasing physical performance capacity. *Biology of Sport* 12: 197-212.

Pauletto, P., and Strumia, E. 1996. Clinical experience with creatine phosphate therapy. In *Creatine and creatine phosphate: Scientific and clinical perspectives,* ed. M.A. Conway and J.F. Clark, pp. 185-198. San Diego: Academic Press.

Pearson, D.R., Hamby, D.G., Russell, W., and Harris, T. 1998. Chronic effects of creatine monohydrate on strength and power. In *Journal of Strength and Conditioning Research* 12: 276. (abstract).

Peeters, B.M., Lantz, C.D., and Mayhew, J.L. 1999. Effect of oral creatine monohydrate and creatine phosphate supplementation on maximal strength indices, body composition, and blood pressure. *Journal of Strength and Conditioning Research.* 13:3-9.

Peyrebrune, M.C., Nevill, M.E., Donaldson, F.J., and Cosford, D.J. 1998. The effects of oral creatine supplementation on performance in single and repeated sprint swimming. *Journal of Sports Sciences* 16: 271-279.

Pirola, V., Pisani, L., and Teruzzi, P. 1991. Evaluation of the recovery of muscular trophicity in aged patients with femoral fractures treated with creatine phosphate and physiokinesitherapy. *Clinica Terapeutica* 139: 115-119.

Plisk, S.S., and Kreider, R.B. 1999. Creatine controversy? *Strength and Conditioning* 21: 14-23.

Podewils, L.J. Effect of creatine supplementation on exercise performance in the heat among college aged males. Master's thesis, San Diego State University, San Diego, CA.

Poortmans, J.R., Auquier, H., Renaut, V., Durussel, A., Saugy, M., and Brisson, G.R. 1997. Effect of short-term creatine supplementation on renal responses in men. *European Journal of Applied Physiology* 76: 566-567.

Poortmans, J.R., and Francaux, M. 1999. Long-term oral creatine supplements do not impair renal function in healthy athletes. *Medicine and Science in Sports and Exercise* 31(5): In press. (abstract).

Poortmans, J.R., and Francaux, M. 1998. Renal dysfunction accompanying oral creatine supplements. *Lancet* 352: 233-234.

Prevost, M.C., Nelson, A.G., and Morris, G.S. 1997. Creatine supplementation enhances intermittent work performance. *Research Quarterly for Exercise and Sport* 68: 233-240.

Pritchard, N.R., and Kaira, P.A. 1998. Renal dysfunction accompanying oral supplements. *Lancet* 351: 1252-1253.

Pulido, S.M., Passaquin, A.C., Leijendekker, W.J., Challet, C., Wallimann, T., and Ruegg, U.T. 1998. Creatine supplementation improves intracellular Ca^{2+} handling and survival in mdx skeletal muscle cells. *FEBS Letters* 439: 357-362.

Radda, G.K. 1996. Control of energy metabolism during muscle metabolism. *Diabetes* 45: S88-S92.

Ransom, J., Kreider, R., Hunt, J., Melton, C., Rasmussen, C., Stroud, T., Cantler, E., Almada, A., and Milnor, P. 1999. Effects of creatine supplementation during training on markers of catabolism and muscle and liver enzymes. *Medicine and Science in Sports and Exercise* 31(5): In press. (abstract).

Rasmussen, C., Kreider, R., Ransom, J., Hunt, J., Melton, C., Stroud, T., Cantler, E., Almada, A., and Milnor, P. 1999. Creatine supplementation during pre-season football training does not affect fluid or electrolyte status. *Medicine and Science in Sports and Exercise* 31(5): In press. (abstract).

Rawson, E.S., Clarkson, P.M., and Melanson, E.L. 1998. The effects of oral creatine supplementation on body mass, isometric strength, and isokinetic performance in older individuals. *Medicine and Science in Sports and Exercise* 30: S140. (abstract).

Redondo, D.R., Dowling, E.A., Graham, B.L., Almada, A.L., and Williams, M.H. 1996. The effect of oral creatine monohydrate supplementation on running velocity. *International Journal of Sport Nutrition* 6: 213-221.

Rossiter, H.B., Cannell, E.R., and Jakeman, P.M. 1996. The effect of oral creatine supplementation on the 1000-m performance of competitive rowers. *Journal of Sports Sciences* 14: 175-179.

Ruden, T.M., Parcell, A.C., Ray, M.L., Moss, K.A., Semler, J.L., Sharp, R.L., Rolfs, G.W., and King, D.S. 1996. Effects of oral creatine supplementation on performance and muscle metabolism during maximal exercise. *Medicine and Science in Sports and Exercise* 28: S81. (abstract).

Sahlin, K. 1986. Metabolic changes limiting muscle performance. In *Biochemistry of exercise VI,* ed. B. Saltin, pp. 323-343. Champaign, IL: Human Kinetics.

Sahlin, K. 1998. Anaerobic metabolism, acid-base balance, and muscle fatigue during high intensity exercise. In *Oxford textbook of sports medicine,* ed. M. Harries, C. Williams, W.D. Stanish, and L.J. Micheli, pp. 69-76. Oxford: Oxford University Press.

Saks, V.A., Stepanov, V., Jaliashvili, I.V., Konerev, E.A., Kryzkanovsky, S.A., and Strumia, E. 1996. Molecular and cellular mechanisms of action for the cardioprotective and therapeutic role of creatine phosphate. In *Creatine and creatine phosphate: Scientific and clinical perspectives,* ed. M.A. Conway and J.F. Clark, pp. 91-114. San Diego: Academic Press.

Saks, V.A. 1996. Cardiac energetics: Compartmentation of creatine kinase and regulation of oxidative phosphorylation. In *Creatine and creatine phosphate: Scientific and clinical perspectives,* ed. M.A. Conway and J.F. Clark, pp. 65-78. San Diego: Academic Press.

Saks, V.A., Bobkov, Y.G., and Strumia, E., eds. 1987. *Creatine phosphate: Biochemistry, pharmacology, and clinical efficiency.* Torino: Edizioni Minerva Medica.

Saks, V.A., Rosenshtraukh, L.V., Smirnov, V.N., and Chazov, E.I. 1978. Role of creatine phosphokinase in cellular function and metabolism. *Canadian Journal of Physiology and Pharmacology* 56: 691-706.

Saks, V.A., and Strumia, E. 1993. Phosphocreatine: molecular and cellular aspects of the mechanism of cardioprotective action. *Current Therapeutic Research* 53: 565-598.

Saks, V.A., and Ventura-Clapier, R. 1992. Biochemical organization of energy metabolism in muscle. *Journal of Biochemical Organization* 1: 9-29.

Satolli, F., and Marchesi, G. 1989. Creatine phosphate in the rehabilitation of patients with muscle hypnotrophy [sic] of the lower extremity. *Current Therapeutic Research* 46: 67-73.

Schaufelberger, M., and Swedberg, K. 1998. Is creatine supplementation helpful for patients with chronic heart failure? *European Heart Journal* 19: 533-534.

Schneider, D.A., McDonough, P.J., Fadel, P.J., and Berwick, J.P. 1997. Creatine supplementation and the total work performed during 15-s and 1-min bouts of maximal cycling. *Australian Journal of Science and Medicine in Sports* 29: 65-68.

Schneider, K., Hervig, L., Ensign, W.Y., Prusaczyk, W.K., and Goforth, H.W. 1998. Use of supplements by U.S. Navy Seals. *Medicine and Science in Sports and Exercise* 30: S60. (abstract).

Sherman, W.M., and Lamb, D.R. 1995. Proceedings of the Gatorade Sports Science Institute Conference on Nutritional Ergogenic Aids. *International Journal of Sport Nutrition* 5: Sii-S131.

Sipilä, I., Rapola, J., Simell, O., and Vannas, A. 1981. Supplementary creatine as a treatment for gyrate atrophy of the choroid and retina. *New England Journal of Medicine* 304: 867-870.

SKW Trostberg. 1998. SKW Trostberg AG announces patent enforcement action, exposes inferior products and introduces Creapure™ brand creatine products. Memorandum, 15 July.

Smart, N.A., McKenzie, S.G., Nix, L.M., Baldwin, S.E., Page, K., Wade, D., and Hampson, P.K. 1998. Creatine supplementation does not improve repeat sprint performance in soccer players. *Medicine and Science in Sports and Exercise* 30: S140. (abstract).

Smith, J.C., Stephens, D.P., Hall, E.L., Jackson, A.W., and Earnest, C.P. 1998a. Effect of oral creatine ingestion on parameters of the work rate-time relationship and time to exhaustion in high-intensity cycling. *European Journal of Applied Physiology* 77: 360-365.

Smith, S.A., Montain, S.J., Matott, R.P., Zientara, G.P., Jolesz, F.A., and Fielding, R.A. 1998b. Creatine supplementation and age influence muscle metabolism during exercise. *Journal of Applied Physiology* 85: 1349-1356.

Snow, R.J., McKenna, M.J., Selig, S.E., Kemp, J., Stathis, C.G., and Zhao, S. 1998. Effect of creatine supplementation on sprint exercise performance and muscle metabolism. *Journal of Applied Physiology* 84: 1667-1673.

Söderlund, K., Balsom, P.D., and Ekblom, B. 1994. Creatine supplementation and high intensity exercise: Influence on performance and muscle metabolism. *Clinical Science* 87 (Suppl.): 120-121.

Spriet, L. 1995. Caffeine and performance. *International Journal of Sports Nutrition* 5: S84-S99.

Stevenson, S.W., and Dudley, G.A. 1998. Creatine supplementation and resistance exercise. *Journal of Strength and Conditioning Research* 12: 278. (abstract).

Stöckler, S., and Hanefeld, F. 1997. Guanidinoacetate methyltransferase deficiency: A newly recognized inborn error of creatine biosynthesis. *Wiener Klinische Wochenschrift* 109(3): 86-88.

Stöckler, S., Hanefeld, F., and Frahm, J. 1996a. Creatine replacement therapy in guanidinoacetate methyltransferase deficiency, a novel inborn error of metabolism. *Lancet* 348: 789-790.

Stöckler, S., Holzbach, U., Hanefeld, F., Marquardt, I., Helms, G., Requart, M., Hänicke, W., and Frahm, J. 1994. Creatine deficiency in the brain: A new, treatable inborn error of metabolism. *Pediatrics Research* 36: 409-413.

Stöckler, S., Isbrandt, D., Hanefeld, F., Schmidt, B., and von Figura, K. 1996b. Guanidinoacetate methyltransferase deficiency: The first inborn error of creatine metabolism in man. *American Journal of Human Genetics* 58: 914-922.

Stöckler, S., Marescau, B., De Deyn, P.P., Trijbels, J.M., and Hanefeld, F. 1997. Guanidino compounds in guanidinoacetate methyltransferase deficiency, a new inborn error of creatine synthesis. *Metabolism* 46: 1189-1193.

Stone, M.H., Sanborn, K., Smith, L., O'Bryant, H.S., Hoke, T., Utter, A., Johnson, R.L., Boros, R., Hruby, J., Pierce, K., Stone, M.E., and Garner, B. 1999. Effects of in-season (5 weeks) creatine and pyruvate supplementation on anaerobic performance and body composition in American football players. *International Journal of Sport Nutrition*: In press.

Stout, J.R., Echerson, J., Noonan, D., Moore, G., and Cullen, D. 1999. Effects of creatine supplementation on exercise performance and fat-free weight in football players during training. *Nutrition Research* 19: 217-225.

Strauss, G. 1998. 1 in 3 pro sports teams say "no" to creatine. *USA Today,* 4 June: News, 1A.

Strauss, G., and Mihoces, G. 1998. Jury still out on creatine use. *USA Today,* 4 June, C1-C2.

Stroud, M.A., Holliman, D., Bell, D., Green, A.L., Macdonald, I., and Greenhaff, P.L. 1994. Effect of oral creatine supplementation on respiratory gas exchange and blood lactate accumulation during steady-state incremental treadmill exercise and recovery in man. *Clinical Science* 87: 707-710.

Syllum-Rapoport, I., Daniel, A., and Rapoport, S. 1980. Creatine transport into red blood cells. *Acta Biologica et Medica Germanica* 39: 771-779.

Syrotuik, D.G., Bell, G.J., Burnham, R., Sim, L.L., Calvert, R.A., and MacLean, I.M. 1998. Absolute and relative strength performance following creatine monohydrate supplementation combined with periodized resistance training. *Journal of Strength and Conditioning Research* 12: 278. (abstract).

Tarnopolsky, M. and Martin, J. 1999. Creatine monohydrate increases strength in patients with neuromuscular disease. *Neurology* 52: 854-7.

Tarnopolsky, M.A., Roy, B.D., and MacDonald, J.R. 1997. A randomized, controlled trial of creatine monohydrate in patients with mitochondrial cytopathies. *Muscle and Nerve* 20: 1502-1509.

Terrillion, K.A., Kolkhorst, F.W., Dolgener, F.A., and Joslyn, S.J. 1997. The effect of creatine supplementation on two 700-m maximal running bouts. *International Journal of Sport Nutrition* 7: 138-143.

Tesch, P.A., Colliander, E.B., and Kaiser, P. 1986. Muscle metabolism during intense, heavy-resistance exercise. *European Journal of Applied Physiology* 55: 362-366.

Theodoru, A.S., Cooke, C.B., King, R.F.G.J., and Duckette, R. 1998. The effect of combined carbohydrate and creatine ingestion on anaerobic performance. *Medicine and Science in Sports and Exercise* 30: S272. (abstract).

Thompson, C.H., Kemp, G.J., Sanderson, A.L., Dixon, R.M., Styles, P., Taylor, D.J., and Radda, G.K. 1996. Effect of creatine on aerobic and anaerobic metabolism in skeletal muscle in swimmers. *British Journal of Sports Medicine* 30: 222-225.

Thorensen, E., McMillam, J., Guion, K., and Joyner, B. 1998. The effect of creatine supplementation on repeated sprint performance. *Journal of Strength and Conditioning Research* 12: 278. (abstract).

Toler, S.M. 1997. Creatine is an ergogen for anaerobic exercise. *Nutrition Reviews* 55: 21-23.

USA Today Editorial. 1998. "Natural" doesn't equal safe, especially in pills and potions. *USA Today,* 30 April: News, 14A.

Vanakoski, J., Kosunen, V., Meririnne, E., and Seppala, T. 1998. Creatine and caffeine in anaerobic and aerobic exercise: Effects on physical performance and pharmacokinetic considerations. *International Journal of Clinical Pharmacology and Therapeutics* 36: 258-262.

Vandenberghe, K., Van Hecke, P., Van Leemputte, M., Vanstapel, F., and Hespel, P. 1999. Phosphocreatine Resynthesis is not affected by creatine loading. *Medicine and Science in Sports and Exercise* 31: 236-242.

Vandenberghe, K., Gillis, N., Van Leemputte, M., Van Hecke, P., Vanstapel, F., and Hespel, P. 1996a. Caffeine counteracts the ergogenic action of muscle creatine loading. *Journal of Applied Physiology* 80: 452-457.

Vandenberghe, K., Goris, M., Van Hecke, P., Van Leemputte, M., Vangerven, L., and Hespel, P. 1996b. Prolonged creatine intake facilitates the effects of strength training on intermittent exercise capacity. *Insider* 4(3): 1-2.

Vandenberghe, K., Goris, M., Van Hecke, P., Van Leemputte, M., Van Gerven, L., and Hespel, P. 1997a. Long-term creatine intake is beneficial to muscle performance during resistance training. *Journal of Applied Physiology* 83: 2055-2063.

Vandenberghe, K., Van Hecke, P., Van Leemputte, M., Vanstapel, F., and Hespel, P. 1997b. Inhibition of muscle phosphocreatine resynthesis by caffeine after creatine loading. *Medicine and Science in Sports and Exercise* 29: S249. (abstract).

van Deursen, J., Heerschap, A., Oerlemans, F., Ruitenbeek, W., Jap, P., ter Laak, H., and Wieringa, B. 1993. Skeletal muscles of mice deficient in muscle creatine kinase lack burst activity. *Cell* 74: 621-631.

van Leemputte, M., Vandenberghe, K., and Hespel, P. 1999. Shortening of muscle relaxation time after creatine loading. *Journal of Applied Physiology* 86: 840-844.

Vannas-Sulonen, K., Sipilä, I., Vannas, A., Simell, O., and Rapola, J. 1985. Gyrate atrophy of the choroid and retina. *Ophthalmology* 92: 1719-1727.

Viru, M., Ööpik, V., Nurmekivi, A., Medijainen, L., Timpmann, S., and Viru, A. 1994. Effect of creatine intake on the performance capacity in middle-distance runners. *Coaching and Sport Science Journal* 1: 31-36.

Volek, J.S. 1997. Creatine supplementation and its possible role in improving physical performance. *ACSM Health Fitness Journal* 1(4): 23-29.

Volek, J.S., Boetes, M., Bush, J.A., Putukian, M., Sebastianelli, W.J., and Kraemer, W.J. 1997a. Response of testosterone and cortisol concentrations to high-intensity resistance exercise following creatine supplementation. *Journal of Strength and Conditioning Research* 11: 182-187.

Volek, J.S., Duncan, N.D., Mazzetti, S.A., Staron, R.S., Putukian, M., Gómez, A.L., Pearson, D.R., Fink, W.J., and Kraemer, W.J. 1999. Performance and muscle fiber adaptations to creatine supplementation and heavy resistance training. *Medicine and Science in Sports and Exercise:* 31. In press.

Volek, J.S., and Kraemer, W.J. 1996. Creatine supplementation: Its effect on human muscular performance and body composition. *Journal of Strength and Conditioning Research* 10: 200-210.

Volek, J.S., Kraemer, W.J., Bush, J.A., Boetes, M., Incledon, T., Clark, K.L., and Lynch, J.M. 1997b. Creatine supplementation enhances muscular performance during high-intensity resistance exercise. *Journal of the American Dietetic Association* 97: 765-770.

Vukovich, M.D., and Michaelis, J. 1999. Effect of two different creatine supplementation products on muscular strength and power. *Sports Medicine, Training, and Rehabilitation* 8: 369-383.

Wadler, G., and Hainline, B. 1989. *Drugs and the athlete.* Philadelphia: Davis.

Walker, J.B. 1960a. Metabolic control of creatine biosynthesis I: Effect of dietary creatine. *Journal of Biological Chemistry* 235: 2357-2361.

Walker, J.B. 1960b. Metabolic control of creatine biosynthesis II: Restoration of transamidinase activity following creatine repression. *Journal of Biological Chemistry* 236: 493-498.

Walker, J.B. 1979. Creatine: Biosynthesis, regulation, and function. *Advances in Enzymology* 50: 177-242.

Walters, P.H., and Olrich, T.W. 1998. The effect of creatine supplementation on strength performance. *Journal of Strength and Conditioning Research* 12: 279. (abstract).

Warber, J.P., Patton, J.F., Tharion, W.J., Montain, S.J., Mello, R.P., and Lieberman, H.R. 1998. Effects of creatine monohydrate supplementation on physical performance. *FASEB Journal* 12: A1040. (abstract).

Whipp, B.J., and Mahler, M. 1980. Dynamics of pulmonary gas exchange during exercise. In *Pulmonary gas exchange, Vol. II: Organism and environment,* ed. J.B. West, pp. 33-96. New York: Academic Press.

Whittingham, T.S., and Lipton, P. 1981. Cerebral synaptic transmission during anoxia is protected by creatine. *Journal of Neurochemistry* 37: 1618-1621.

Williams, M.H. 1974. *Drugs and athletic performance.* Springfield, IL: Charles C Thomas.

Williams, M.H. 1985. *Nutritional aspects of human physical and athletic performance.* Springfield, IL: Charles C Thomas.

Williams, M.H. 1994. The use of nutritional ergogenic aids in sports: Is it an ethical issue? *International Journal of Sport Nutrition* 4: 120-131.

Williams, M.H. 1999. *Nutrition for health, fitness and sport.* Dubuque, IA. WCB/McGraw-Hill.

Williams, M.H., and Branch, J.D. 1998. Creatine supplementation and exercise performance: An update. *Journal of the American College of Nutrition* 17: 216-234.

Wilson, D.F. 1994. Factors affecting the rate and energetics of mitochondrial oxidative phosphorylation. *Medicine and Science in Sports and Exercise* 26: 37-43.

Wood, K.K., Zabik, R.M., Dawson, M.L., and Frye, P.A. 1998. The effects of creatine monohydrate supplementation on strength, lean body mass, and circumferences in male weightlifters. *Medicine and Science in Sports and Exercise* 30: S272. (abstract).

Wyss, M., Febler, S., Skladal, D., Koller, A., Kremser, C., and Sperl, W. 1998. The therapeutic potential of oral creatine supplementation in muscle disease. *Medical Hypotheses* 51: 333-336.

Zehnder, M., Rico-Sanz, J., Kuhne, G., Dambach, M., Buchli, R., and Boutellier, U. 1998. Muscle phosphocreatine and glycogen concentrations in humans after creatine and glucose polymer supplementation measured noninvasively by ^{31}P and ^{13}C-MRS. *Medicine and Science in Sports and Exercise* 30: S264. (abstract).

Ziegenfuss, T., Gales, D., Felix, S., Straehle, S., Klemash, K., Konrath, D., and Lemon, P.W.R. 1998a. Performance benefits following a five day creatine loading procedure persist for at least four weeks. *Medicine and Science in Sports and Exercise* 30: S265. (abstract).

Ziegenfuss, T., Lemon, P.W.R., Rogers, M.R., Ross, R., and Yarasheski, K.E. 1997. Acute creatine ingestion: Effects on muscle volume, anaerobic power, fluid volumes, and protein turnover. *Medicine and Science in Sports and Exercise* 29: S127. (abstract).

Ziegenfuss, T.N., Lowery, L.M., and Lemon, P.W.R. 1998b. Acute fluid volume changes in men during three days of creatine supplementation. *Journal of Exercise Physiology*$_{online}$ 1(3): 1-9. **http://www.css.edu/users/tboone2/asep/jan13.htm.**

Index

About the Authors

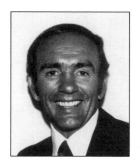

Melvin Williams, PhD, is Eminent Scholar Emeritus in the Department of Exercise Science, Physical Education, and Recreation at Old Dominion University. He has conducted research on various ergogenic aids for over 30 years and has published numerous original research studies and review articles.

Author of *The Ergogenics Edge* (Human Kinetics, 1998), Dr. Williams also wrote the definitive college text, *Nutrition for Fitness and Sport*, now in its fifth edition. He is also the founding editor of the *International Journal of Sport Nutrition*. Dr. Williams is a Fellow of the American College of Sports Medicine (ACSM) and a member of the American Alliance for Health, Physical Education, Recreation and Dance. Dr. Williams lives in Norfolk, Virginia.

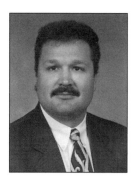

Richard B. Kreider, PhD, is associate professor, assistant department chair, and director of the Exercise and Sport Nutrition Laboratory in the Department of Human Movement Sciences and Education at the University of Memphis. He has focused his research efforts on ergogenic aids and human physical performance and has conducted numerous studies on creatine supplementation.

Editor of the popular reference, *Overtraining in Sport* (Human Kinetics, 1998), Dr. Kreider has published more than 100 research articles and abstracts in scientific journals. He is a Fellow of the ACSM and the research digest editor for the *International Journal of Sport Nutrition*. Dr. Kreider lives in Bartlett, Tennessee.

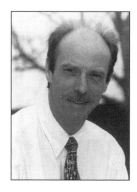

J. David Branch, PhD, is assistant professor of exercise science at Old Dominion University. He has conducted several studies involving ergogenic aids, including the effects of creatine supplementation on women.

Since 1980 Dr. Branch has been supervisor of Bicycle Ergometer Graded Exercise Testing for the South Carolina State Law Enforcement Health/Fitness Screening Program. He has also served as codirector of a fitness and cardiac rehabilitation center.

Dr. Branch is a Fellow of the ACSM and has been widely published. He lives in Norfolk, Virginia.

Related Books by Human Kinetics

The Ergogenics Edge
Mel Williams, PhD
1998 • Paperback • 328 pp • Item PWIL0545
ISBN 0-88011-545-9 • $17.95 ($26.95 Canadian)

For more than 30 years, Mel Williams has researched and explained the nutritional, pharmacological, psychological, and physiological ergogenics that should and should not be used in sports. *The Ergogenics Edge* provides information on a wide variety of ergogenics and analyzes their positive and negative effects on sports performance factors (SPFs).

Overtraining in Sport
Richard B. Kreider, PhD, Andrew C. Fry, PhD, and Mary L. O'Toole, PhD, Editors
1998 • Hardback • 416 pp • Item BKRE0563
ISBN 0-88011-563-7 • $45.00 ($67.50 Canadian)

Overtraining in Sport is the first comprehensive text on the physiological, biomedical, and psychological aspects of overtraining and overreaching in sport. Thirty-three leading researchers contribute 17 chapters to this multidisciplinary review of recent findings.

The Steroids Game
Charles Yesalis and Virginia Cowart
1998 • Paperback • 216 pp • Item PYES0494
ISBN 0-88011-494-0 • $16.95 ($24.95 Canadian)

The Steroids Game cuts through the hype and misinformation surrounding the use of anabolic steroids with solid facts and expert commentary on a drug problem that has filtered its way into every level of sports.

To request more information or to order, U.S. customers call 1-800-747-4457, e-mail us at humank@hkusa.com, or visit our website at www.humankinetics.com. Persons outside the U.S. can contact us via our website or use the appropriate telephone number, postal address, or e-mail address shown in the front of this book.

Human Kinetics
The Information Leader in Physical Activity